THE 7-DAY HEALTHY HEART DIET

G

GALVAN!ZED
Media

This book proposes a program of diet and exercise recommendations for the reader to follow. However, you should consult a qualified medical professional (and, if you are pregnant, your ob-gyn) before starting this or any other diet or fitness program. Please seek your doctor's advice before making any decisions that affect your health or extreme changes in your diet, particularly if you suffer from any medical condition or have any symptom that may require treatment. As with any diet or exercise program, if at any time you experience discomfort, stop immediately and consult your physician.

Mention of specific companies, organizations, or authorities in this book does not imply endorsement by the author or publisher, nor does mention of specific companies, organizations, or authorities imply that they endorse this book, its author, or the publisher.

Distributed by Simon & Schuster

ISBN 9781940358383
Ebook ISBN 9781940358390

Printed in the United States of America on acid-free paper.

Design by Andy Turnbull

THE 7-DAY HEALTHY HEART DIET

The Science-Based Plan To Lose Belly Fat And Get You on the Path to Greater Health

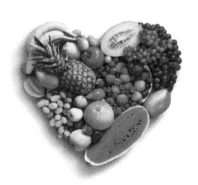

BY JULIE STEWART
AND THE EDITORS OF

Eat This, Not That!®

Contents

Why It's Time to Invest in Your Heart Health

Heart disease is a silent killer. Prevent it now by making some simple lifestyle changes.

LYNNE TROELSTRUP and her husband, Mike, were walking around their Florida neighborhood one evening when she felt a pang of nausea. She figured it was food poisoning—after all, she'd wolfed down a burger earlier that night as she was waiting for a client at work. But as her stomach started to turn over and over, Troelstrup felt so much pain that she had to stop and sit in her driveway. She asked her husband to call 9-1-1.

The paramedics arrived and strapped Troelstrup to a stretcher, and within minutes, everything went dark. Troelstrup didn't have food poisoning. She was suffering from a widowmaker, a heart attack that occurs when the heart's left coronary artery is severely blocked, choking the heart of vital blood flow. Technically called an ST-segment elevation myocardial infarction (STEMI), the widowmaker gets its nickname honestly—it's among the deadliest of heart attacks.

Troelstrup's heart stopped for four minutes. She was transported to the hospital and had to be defibrillated eight times because just as quickly as her pulse would return it would disappear again. Her skin was turning chalky white. Her feet were turning blue. Medical professionals told Troelstrup's husband there was only a two percent chance she would survive, and that even if she did she might have permanent brain damage because her brain was deprived of blood flow for so long.

"You never think it's going to happen to you," says Troelstrup, who is in her 50s. "I never thought I would have a heart attack, but when it happens to you, everything changes."

Fortunately, doctors were able to remove the clot with angioplasty, and after a 14-day hospital stay, she went home.

In the two years since, she has stayed steadfastly committed to following a Mediterranean-style diet that's low in sodium and trans fats and to walking every day. The lifestyle changes are working. When Troelstrup meets new doctors, they are shocked to learn that she nearly died from a heart attack just a couple of years ago. Her advice?

"Get healthy before something happens to you," she says. "Don't take your life and lifestyle for granted."

✳ ✳ ✳

LYNNE TROELSTRUP SHARES HER STORY WITH US BECAUSE SHE wants you to learn from her experience and take action to improve your health now, while you're still healthy. Don't wait for heart trouble to start taking better care of your body because heart attack symptoms may never give you the benefit of a timely warning. Heart disease is the leading cause of premature death for men and women in America, according to the Centers for Disease Control and Prevention, and every year, about 735,000 Americans have a heart attack.

Says Troelstrup: "You don't want to have that feeling I had in my driveway."

AND YOU DON'T HAVE TO!

"Make no mistake—with very rare, genetically induced exception, coronary artery disease doesn't need to develop," said preventive medicine specialist David Katz, MD, during a panel discussion addressing the powerful influence of diet on heart health at the American College of Cardiology conference in 2018. Coronary artery disease, which led to Troelstrup's heart attack, occurs when the arteries harden and become narrowed by a buildup of plaque on their inner walls (atherosclerosis), reducing blood flow and triggering a potentially life-ending clot. "The distal, or root causes, are a lifestyle subordinate to the dictates of culture—a culture

$329.7 billion

The annual direct and indirect cost of cardiovascular disease and stroke in the United States, according to the American Heart Association.

that runs on Dunkin'; peddles multicolored marshmallows as part of a complete breakfast; and conflates the Olympics with a trifecta of fast food, junk food, and sugar-sweetened beverages," writes Katz, author of the book *Disease-Proof* and a member of the Eat This, Not That! board of advisors.

Decades of research have given us a formula for preventing heart disease and other health problems. Katz says: "Fully 80 percent of all chronic disease associated with premature death around the world is preventable with uncontroversial knowledge we already have."

It's simple. It's straightforward. It's all about our food.

But obviously, prevention doesn't happen with a simple bite of an apple, or we would all be skinny marathon runners. It takes sustained effort and commitment. But if you start making lifestyle changes of the sort that Troelstrup has made, you'll begin reducing your risks of disease and elevating your health immediately.

" Make no mistake—with very rare, genetically induced exception—coronary artery disease does not need to develop."

—DAVID KATZ, MD, AUTHOR OF *DISEASE-PROOF*

Look, you change the oil in your car regularly, right? You check your bank balance before you write a big check so you're certain it won't bounce, don't you? You clean the lint from that flexible exhaust tube on your clothes dryer twice a year to prevent a fire. (You do, don't you?) All of those actions prevent a problem: your engine seizing up, your check bouncing, your house burning down. So why not pay more attention to something that's way more important than even those important things? Your heart and arteries deserve TLC.

We wrote this book to encourage you to press the pause button on all the things in life that are keeping you from taking charge of your health. The 7-Day Healthy Heart Diet is a one-week step-by-step plan that moves heart health to the top of your to-do list. The information here will help you adopt some key practices that you can easily maintain for the rest of your life. You have to start somewhere, and this is an excellent place to begin because our program puts healthy living on autopilot, with little reminders that keep you on track until they become ingrained in your lifestyle and become a natural part of how you live your life. Then, you won't have to think about them.

You know that little mileage sticker on the windshield that reminds you when it's time for an oil change? The Healthy Heart Diet is similar, but our "sticker" reminds you to Eat This for lunch, Not That! It prompts you to fill a tumbler of lemon water to drink at your work desk instead of a half gallon of sweet tea or soda. It helps you recognize just how much sugar, sodium, and industrial trans fats you are unwittingly ingesting every day, and it gives you a practical plan to stop the assault of the salt. The 7-Day Healthy Heart Diet program sets up a realistic plan to build exercise into your day. We know you're busy; our plan understands and gives you a schedule that helps you fit it into your day.

WHAT TO EXPECT

As we've said, the 7-Day Healthy Heart Diet won't be successful without your buy-in and hard work. Nothing worthwhile comes from a snap of your fingers. You must want to change your life and find the discipline to do it. But in one week on this plan, you'll reap some big, noticeable rewards that'll keep you motivated to adopt the healthy heart lifestyle for life. Here's what you can expect to happen in 7 days—and beyond:

- You'll lose weight to begin taking some of the extra strain off your heart.

- You'll strengthen your heart and keep your arteries flexible and healthy.

- You'll improve your blood pressure reading and cholesterol levels, and you'll reduce your risk of type 2 diabetes by up to 60 percent.

- You'll start to whittle away at your middle, the visceral belly fat that's the cause of so many of our lifestyle-created diseases.

- Over time, you'll save tons of money on health-care costs, according to research published in the medical journal *Circulation*.

- You'll become healthier from head to toe and likely live a longer, more active, and happier life.

It all sounds very good, right? It's what you want. It's what we all want. But are those valuable assets enough to get you to take the first critical steps outlined in Chapter

1? We hope so. But let's be sure. For some extra motivation that we believe will resonate with you, put down this book for a moment and find a photograph of your family. Take a look at the smiling faces and ask yourself what they would lose by losing you to a heart attack, heart failure, or a stroke.

You see, protecting your heart is no selfish endeavor. You are doing it for the people who love you and rely on you, for the people you love. Keep those others in mind as you begin focusing deliberately on your own well-being.

Now, indulge us in one other request: Turn the page and fill out the simple family health chart you'll find there. There's room for Mom and Dad, your grandparents, and your siblings. Fill it out as best you can, listing the age of any diagnosis. The chart could be a window into your future health. Bring it to your next doctor's checkup. Use it make yourself and your doctor aware of potential hereditary disease risks so you can take the appropriate preventive action now.

Log Your Family Heart Health History
* Bring to your physician.

FAMILY MEMBER	HEART DISEASE	HEART ATTACK	DIABETES	STROKE
Mother				
Father				
Sibling				
Sibling				
Sibling				
Sibling				
Sibling				
Maternal grandmother				
Maternal grandfather				
Paternal grandmother				
Paternal grandfather				

The 7-Day Healthy Heart Diet at a Glance

We broke a lifestyle overhaul into six simple (and fun!) steps.

LBERT EINSTEIN said, "If you can't explain it, you don't know it well enough." Isn't it the truth? You know what K.I.S.S. stands for, right? Not the '70s' costumed rock band, but the design principle: Keep It Simple Stupid? Same concept: Simple is always better than complicated when you are trying to remember something important.

Take poison ivy, for example: If you remember the simple phrase "Leaves of three, let it be," you'll avoid touching any plants that may give you an oozing rash. If you're trying to recall the phases of mitosis (cell division) for your biology exam, saying to yourself the mnemonic **I propose men are toads** may help you remember—**i**nterphase, **p**rophase, **m**etaphase, **a**naphase, **t**elophase. Don't you feel smarter already?

OK, you get our point about simple. It works. That's why we've taken something as complicated as cardiovascular health and boiled it down to a simple plan of *more this, less that*—key points you can count on your fingers, even if you only have six fingers!

MORE THIS:
1. PLANTS
2. EXERCISE
3. HEALTHY FATS
4. SLEEP

LESS THAT:
5. SALT
6. SUGAR

If you remember every day to:
1. Eat more plants
2. Exercise your heart
3. Add hunger-satisfying healthy fats to your meals
4. Sleep 7 or more hours a night
5. Reduce sodium in your foods
6. Avoid added sugars and processed carbohydrates—you will automatically lose weight and dramatically improve your heart health. And you can make these action items a daily occurence in 7 days or less. Let's review them:

Step 1: Pile your plate with plants

The term "superfood" gets thrown around a lot, but the truth is that this word shouldn't only apply to rare berries harvested from a remote corner of the world. Many plant foods have superpowers because they contain helpful compounds, including vitamins, minerals, and antioxidants that tamp down inflammation or counteract harmful oxidative stress.

When you hear the word "inflammation," you might imagine a swollen pimple or an ankle that that feels hot and sore after you turned it during a run. The truth is that our immune systems produce inflammatory molecules all the time. That's OK to a point, but when you have *too much* inflammation, your heart and other body parts can become collateral damage. There are many things that trigger inflammation, and some foods, such as table sugar, fried foods, and refined flours, are among the ones that do. In a study in the *International Journal of Cardiology*, people with the most inflammatory eating patterns were 37 to 50 percent more likely to have cardiovascular risk factors than people with healthier eating habits.

To eat more anti-inflammatory nutrients, most doctors and dieticians recommend a "plant-based" diet. But that doesn't mean you have to go vegan—you just need to pile your plate with more whole grains, fruits, vegetables, legumes, and nuts than you usually do. Many traditional diets, from the Mediterranean diet to the Nordic diet, are based on whole, natural, plant-based foods, and scientists who study these diets largely reach a similar conclusion: These styles of eating are far healthier than the typical American diet, which is loaded with saturated fat, low-fiber carbohydrates like added sugars, sodium, and calories. Of course, there are plenty of plant-based foods that *aren't* healthy (potato chips, anyone?), and we'll sort those out, too, in Chapters 5 and 6.

Your Healthy Heart Diet Goal: Eat four to six servings of vegetables, two to four servings of fruits, and one serving of legumes every day. We'll give you delicious recipes in Chapter 10 that make getting that much plant food easy to swallow.

Step 2: Exercise your heart every day

Wait, you say you're busy? Between the job, kids, and your Fortnite addiction, you can't spare time to get to a gym? With our plan, you don't have to. We'll show you ways to build much more movement into your daily activities as well as make time for formal exercise without sacrificing important parts of the rest of your life.

But do know this: Regular exercise is really important for good heart health. You can't get around this one. See, exercise trains your heart to work more efficiently. People who work out hard on a regular basis have lower heart rates and pump more blood with each heartbeat, according to a study review published in the *British Journal of Sports Medicine*. A heart that beats more slowly and recovers more quickly from exertion beats longer.

Exercise may also increase your body's ability to break down fatty molecules that could otherwise clog your arteries. Fit people tend to have less of the kind of inflammation in their bodies that damages their arteries. And of course, exercise burns calories, which means it can help you build more lean muscle and reduce body fat at the same time, complementing the effects of your diet plan.

If your exercise regimen is inconsistent or nonexistent, now is the time to step it up—especially if you spend hours a day sitting at a desk. Researchers in the UK found that the people with the healthiest metabolic markers were those who walked more than 15,000 steps per day or spent more than seven hours per day standing. Scheduled workouts are important, but it's also critical to just move more every day. That means taking the stairs instead of the elevator, walking at lunchtime and after work, and building more physical activity into every day. We offer suggestions and suggest a time-efficient workout in Chapter 4.

Your Healthy Heart Diet Goal: Walk at least 10,000 steps every day—easy to track with your smartphone—and do a mix of aerobic interval training and strength training 5 days a week.

Step 3: Add healthy fats to your meals

Back in the '90s, we were told that fat was bad for our hearts. But the medical community has changed its tune on fat. Yes, certain fats can be harmful to the heart, but other fats are healthful to eat. Many foods rich in fat, from avocados to fish to nuts and more, are proven heart helpers, and we'll show you how to pick the right ones and avoid the problematic ones, such as industrial trans fats and the saturated fats in fried foods.

Look, we love french fries as much as you do, but you should know right now that we're going to ask you to keep the fries to a rare, occasional treat. Fries are just not good for the ol' ticker. A key study in the venerable *Journal of the American Heart Association* made that point clear: It compared men who ate fried food less than once a week to men who ate a lot of fried foods and found that those who indulged in fried fare often were between 24 and 203 percent more likely to develop heart failure.

Frying increases the fat and calorie content of foods, and it has been shown to inhibit an enzyme that would otherwise tamp down oxidation of low-density lipoprotein (LDL) cholesterol, the bad kind. That's important because oxidized LDL particles may be especially damaging to your blood vessels.

Your Healthy Heart Diet Goal: Eliminate fried foods from your diet, or limit fried foods to a once-a-week indulgence. And replace saturated fats with healthier fats like the monounsaturated fat in olive oil. Get about one-third of your daily calories in fat from nutritious, filling sources. We'll show you how to eat the best nuts and seeds, dairy products, fish, meats, and oils and steer clear of bad fats.

Step 4: Sleep 7 hours or more per night

Whether it's pulling all-nighters or sleeping way past the ding of your alarm, an out-of-whack sleep pattern could give you a weary heart. In a study published in *Sleep Medicine,* people who slept just one to four hours per night were 2.4 times more likely to have a cardiovascular condition than those who slept seven to nine hours per night. On the flipside, people who overdid it and slept 10 to 18 hours a night were almost 7.2 times more likely to have a cardiovascular condition than those who got the right amount of shut-eye. The sleep and heart health correlation might be linked by multiple factors, one of which is that people who have trouble sleeping tend to have higher levels of harmful inflammation, suggests research from UCLA. Sure, the number of hours you spend in bed matters, but no surprise, the quality of your sleep is also important.

Of course, the easy part is recognizing that you need more sleep, and the hard part is figuring out how to get it. Fortunately, we have a few easy strategies for you.

Your Healthy Heart Diet Goal: Train yourself to get better-quality sleep and log seven to nine hours per night. You're not dreaming. While we can't stop your kids from waking you up in the middle of the night, we can give you the tools and techniques to improve your sleep (in Chapter 8).

Step 5: Avoid high-sodium foods

You might be surprised to know how much sodium you eat in an average day—about 3,400 milligrams for the average American, according to the American Heart Association. That's more than double the recommended amount. For people with blood pressure trouble, excess salt can be a problem because it may contribute to hypertension. An estimated 80 million Americans have high blood pressure, and left untreated, it can put you at greater risk for heart disease.

You never use a salt shaker, you say? Doesn't matter. You're likely still consuming too much from hidden sources. Nine out of 10 Americans get too much salt, according to new figures released by the Centers for Disease Control and Prevention. And 77 percent of that sodium comes from processed or restaurant foods.

U.S. dietary guidelines suggest we should get less than 2,300 milligrams (mg) of sodium each day. However, if you or someone in your family has a history of high blood pressure, the American Heart Association recommends limiting sodium intake to no more than 1,500 mg a day. Here's another reason to slash the sodium: Salty foods are so palatable that it's easy to overeat them (think potato chips), making them especially problematic for people trying to lose weight.

Your Healthy Heart Diet Goal: Recognize how much salt you're consuming from restaurant and packaged foods and be diligent about avoiding high-sodium foods. That means reading nutrition labels and cooking more of your meals at home. If you limit going out to eat to, say, once a week (once every two weeks would be even better), you'll automatically slash your sodium intake by at least one-third.

Step 6: Eliminate added sugars and processed carbohydrates from your diet

One of the simplest ways to improve your health is to upgrade your approach to eating carbohydrates. Carbs aren't inherently evil—far from it. They are an important part of a healthy diet. After all, vegetables, fruits, and whole grains are all carbs. It's the processed, sugary carbs (like the sugar and refined flour in breads) that you should approach with caution. Refined, simple carbs can contribute to blood sugar spikes, drive cravings through the roof, and increase the body's production of fat.

Added sugars—the sugars dumped into processed foods to sweeten them—are clearly dangerous for your heart. People in a recent study published in *JAMA Internal Medicine* who consumed the lowest amount of added sugar, comprising less than 10 percent of their daily calories, had the lowest risk of dying from cardiovascular disease. In another study, people who consumed 10 to 25 percent of their calories from added sugars were 30 percent more likely to end up dying from heart disease than people who ate less sugar, while those who consumed 25 percent or more of their calories from added sugar were 2.75 times as likely to have ticker trouble. There are many, many reasons why excess sugar is bad for you, and in Chapter 4, we'll help you wean yourself off the sweet stuff.

Refined grains can also be problematic because they lack many of the nutrients that are present in whole grains that can actually help your heart.

Your Healthy Heart Diet Goal: Eat fewer than 6 teaspoons of added sugars per day if you are a woman, 9 teaspoons a day if you are a man. At the same time, minimize refined grains and instead eat three servings of whole grains per day. We'll show you how in Chapter 7.

THE 10-POUND DIFFERENCE

All six steps of our plan will immediately begin doing good things to your cardiovascular system. But there's another key benefit you'll gain: weight loss. These steps do double duty by shedding excess fat *and* reducing your body weight, which will help your heart in a big way. Here's how:

When you carry extra pounds, you burden your heart with baggage. (We'll show you how to find out whether your weight is hurting your heart in Chapter 2.) Extra weight on your frame promotes high blood pressure, high cholesterol, high blood sugar, and harmful inflammation in your body. Fortunately, losing that extra weight—and it doesn't have to be a ton—can help your heart out: In a study from Washington University in St. Louis, people who lost a modest amount of weight—even just 5 percent of their body weight—reduced their blood pressure by an average of 5 points, their non-HDL cholesterol by 16 points, their triglycerides by 18 points, and their fasting blood sugar by 3 milligrams per deciliter.

Sounds good, but what does that all mean? The researchers estimate that these small improvements in health could decrease lifetime risk of cardiovascular disease by about 22 percent. And it's likely that shedding even more weight would reduce risk even more. But let's play it conservatively. Study author Samuel Klein, MD, the William H. Danforth Professor of Medicine and Nutritional Science at Washington University in St. Louis, recommends starting with a goal of just 5 percent weight loss. If you weigh 200 pounds, that means you only need to shed 10 pounds to give your heart huge health benefits. If you're at 168 pounds, the weight of the average American woman, 5 percent is just 8 pounds. You can reach this goal or be well on your way toward it within 7 days on our program.

In the next chapter, we'll detail steps that will help you accelerate your weight loss while strengthening your heart.

Chapter 1 Action Summary

● Fill out your Family Heart Health History (page XIV) and review it with your doctor.

● Create a plan to lose at least 10 pounds in the next several weeks by incorporating the *More This, Less That* steps below into your life this week.

● **Step 1:** Fill your plate with superfoods—four to six servings of vegetables, two to four servings of fruits, and a serving of legumes every day.

● **Step 2:** Exercise. Walk at least 10,000 steps daily, and do a mix of aerobic interval training and strength training 5 days a week.

● **Step 3:** Add healthy monounsaturated fats to satisfy your hunger while reducing the amount of fried foods and saturated fats you eat.

● **Step 4:** Sleep 7 to 9 hours per night.

● **Step 5:** Avoid high-sodium foods by reading nutrition labels, and eating nearly all of your meals at home.

● **Step 6:** Eliminate added sugars and processed carbohydrates.

The 7-Day Healthy Heart

IT'S SIMPLE. Just get *more of this*, and *less of that*, and you'll be on your way to a healthier heart in one week.

1. More Plants

Pile your plate with plants. Load up on leafy greens and add brightly colored vegetables like peppers, tomatoes, and more. Boost your plant-based protein intake with legumes like beans, chickpeas, and peanuts.

2. More Exercise

Exercise your heart every day. If you're not doing anything now, start walking every day at a brisk pace. Build strength and endurance with the recommended workouts in Chapter 4.

3. More Healthy Fats

Add healthy fats to your meals to stay feeling full longer. Get your healthy fats from olive oil, avocado, fatty fish, seeds, and nuts. Reduce your consumption of saturated fats, and eliminate dangerous trans fats.

Diet at a Glance

4. More Sleep

Sleep 7 or more hours per night. Believe it or not, sleep is a major calorie burner. Getting enough sleep reduces cravings for carbs, gives you more energy during the day, and affects your heart health in many ways.

5. Less Sodium

Avoid salty foods. Sodium, like sugars, is lurking hidden in all sorts of foods that you eat daily. Become a sodium sleuth. Search nutrition labels and be aware of high sodium counts in fast foods. While your body requires sodium, most of us get way too much. Our plan will help you avoid overconsumption.

6. Less Sugar

Eliminate added sugars and processed carbohydrates from your diet. Simply eliminating packaged goods such as cookies, cakes, boxed cereals, condiments, and heat-and-serve meals will significantly slash the added sugars in your diet. Be a sugars sleuth by reading nutrition labels.

2

Strip Away Belly Fat, Strip Away Trouble

Learn easy ways to shed those harmful pounds and add to your cardiovascular health.

EOPLE WHO ARE HEAVY can be quite healthy. Big Al might outweigh everyone at the office, but he may boast lower cholesterol numbers than you. The guy in the "Dilly Dilly" T-shirt that's not quite covering his beer gut could surprise you by leaving you in the dust at the local Turkey Trot 5K. Aunt Rose may be borderline obese, but she can still polka like the dance floor is burning.

It's true, you can be fat and still be fit, but that shouldn't lull anyone into a false sense of security when it comes to cardiovascular disease. Carrying extra weight is a significant risk factor even if you currently have no other risk factors, according to a recent British study in the *European Heart Journal* that compared 7,600 people who had had cardiovascular events with 10,000 people who didn't have heart problems. Researchers found that the people who were considered overweight yet healthy still were 26 percent more likely to develop heart disease than their normal-weight peers. What's more, people who had high blood pressure, high cholesterol, and a waist size larger than 37 inches for men and 31 inches for women were more than twice as likely to have heart disease whether they were overweight or normal weight. "Our study shows that people with excess weight who might be classed as 'healthy' haven't yet developed an unhealthy metabolic profile," said study coauthor Ioanna Tzoulaki, an epidemiologist at Imperial College London's School of Public Health in a news release. "That comes later in the timeline, then they have an event, such as a heart attack," she said.

Carrying around extra weight is simply bad for your heart. That's a sobering statement for the 35 percent of American adults whose body mass index (BMI) is between 25 and 30, which puts them in the overweight category, and the 30 percent who are considered obese (with a BMI over 30).

Fortunately, as we learned at the end of the last chapter, you can quickly start to protect your heart by losing even a modest 5 percent of your body weight. You can easily start that in the next 7 days by following the 6-step plan we've designed for you. In this chapter, you'll find useful tips and strategies to help you eat more mindfully and stay motivated; they complement the diet and exercise plan detailed later in the book.

As someone who has fought a fluctuating waistline since childhood, I understand that it can be a struggle to wrap your mind around your body fat and what to do about it. To start, you might wonder: Do *I* need to lose weight, and if so, how much?

Fortunately, there is a simple, free way to find the answer. Grab a tape measure and a calculator. We'll show you how to measure your waist-to-height ratio, which compares how round you are to how tall you are. Several studies suggest that this magic number is a very good indicator of your body composition, and knowing yours will help to motivate you during our program and gauge your progress. In a study published in *Military Medicine*, all soldiers who achieved a waist-to-height ratio of 0.55 or lower also reached the Army's standards for body fat.

Here's how to do measure it: Wrap a cloth tape measure around your abdomen at its smallest point. Round down to the nearest half inch. Repeat two more times and average them. Now divide that number by your height in inches to get your waist-to-height ratio. Generally, you want to keep your waist circumference to less than half your height. If your ratio is 53 percent or more, you're considered overweight. A ratio of 63 percent or more indicates obesity.

A large belly is a risk factor for cardiovascular disease because of the dangerous type of fat that typically resides there—visceral belly fat. Also called "deep fat," it's a particularly active fat that forms around the vital inner organs. It's dangerous because it secretes toxins and fatty acids that are swept up by the bloodstream and dumped into the liver, negatively impacting the production of cholesterol. Research in the journal *Diabetes* also suggests that visceral fat pumps out immune system chemicals called cytokines that can increase the risk of cardiovascular disease by promoting insulin resistance and chronic inflammation.

Your midsection is also home to intrahepatic fat, which wraps around your liver itself. Research published in the *American Journal of Medicine* suggests that visceral fat and intrahepatic fat are more strongly linked with heart-harming risk factors than other types of fat. Study author Michelle Long, MD, an assistant professor of medicine at Boston University Medical Center, says these fat stores can worsen insulin resistance and increase inflammation.

"Fortunately, weight loss, by any mechanism, will help reduce visceral and intrahepatic fat mass," says Dr. Long. "We know that a 5 to 10 percent weight loss can dramatically improve the amount of liver fat, so this is what we target for patients. The goal is to develop a healthy eating lifestyle that is sustainable over the long term."

We want to help you lose weight or maintain a healthy weight, and the diet and exercise suggestions in this book are designed to help you in those efforts. To stay motivated and maximize your results, start practicing these seven slimming habits.

1. Eat with Intention

Perhaps you have heard of mindful eating, a movement that has gained traction over the past few years. The premise is simple: If you eat thoughtfully and enjoy your food, you will find yourself naturally and effortlessly eating less. Scarfing down mass quantities of food isn't just bad for your waistline, after all; it's bad for your heart, too. Researchers at Brigham and Women's Hospital in Boston found that one heavy meal may bump of risk of heart attack by four times in a two-hour window after the feast. To eat more intentionally...

Keep food in the kitchen instead of placing heaping bowls on the table, which encourages overeating. A study in the journal *Obesity* suggests that when a meal is served family-style, people consume 35 percent more. To avoid temptation, keep food on the stove or counter and spoon it out onto plates from there. When going back for seconds requires leaving the table, people tend to consider their hunger levels more carefully.

Turn off your TV and music at mealtime. A study published in the *American Journal of Clinical Nutrition* found that people who ate in front of the TV consumed 10 percent more than they normally would, and it didn't matter if they were watching *The Chew* or *Dancing with the Stars*. A study published in the journal *Appetite* found that people who listened to music while dining ate more food, and it didn't matter the pace or the volume of the music playing. Eating while distracted disrupts your satiety signals, so shutting off your electronics while munching may help you stick to reasonable portions. As you eat, focus on your food and tune in to your feelings of fullness.

Slow down. A study published in the *American Journal of Clinical Nutrition* found that chewing more and eating slowly caused participants to ingest fewer calories. Chewing food more thoroughly simultaneously lowered levels of appetite-stimulating hormones and increased levels of appetite-suppressing hormones, researchers say. To slow down your munching, place your fork on the table in between bites and don't pick it up again until some time after you've swallowed. A study in the *Journal of the American Dietetic Association* found that slow eaters took in 66 fewer calories per meal than their faster-eating peers. And they felt as if they had actually eaten more. While 66 calories might not sound like much, cutting that amount out of every meal could add up to a weight loss of more than 20 pounds a year.

2. Adopt a Weight-Loss Mind-Set

By shifting your outlook and adjusting a few habits, you can increase your odds of success. Start by taking the phrase "rise and shine" literally every morning. Researchers from Northwestern University found that people who were exposed to bright daylight earlier in the day tended to weigh less than those who didn't get sunlight until later. Right after you wake up, open the blinds and let the sunshine in. Or better yet, step outside and enjoy your morning cup of coffee on the front porch.

Next, consider your motivations. Research suggests what motivates you to get in shape can play a role in your success. A 2014 study in the journal *Body Image* looked at 321 college-age women and found that, long-term, those who exercised primarily for appearance-based reasons had a harder time sticking to their fitness plans than those who worked out to maintain their health. In other words, stop envying those fit models on Instagram and instead remember that you and your loved ones are the people who really benefit when you slim down.

Planning is a big part of adopting a weight-loss mind-set. One helpful habit to get into is meal prepping. After a long workweek, the last thing you probably want to do on Sunday is work some more. But taking time to prep some meals for the coming week can work weight-loss wonders. Sunday meal prep is like setting your sneakers out the night before a run; by stocking your fridge with premade options, you're more likely to reach for what's already available the next time you're hungry. And in this case, it'll be something healthy like a grilled chicken rice bowl or a colorful salad. Check Chapter 9 for more tips on how to prep.

3. Pack a Lunch

When you are finished cooking, portion out just enough for your meal, then pack the rest away for "leftovers." The longer your food sits out, the more likely you are to nibble and go back for seconds (or thirds). Same goes for when you're dining out: Ask for a to-go box along with your meal, that way you can pack away the leftovers and won't be tempted to keep eating. It's instant meal prep!

4. Shop Smarter

If you walk mindlessly around the grocery store, you'll have a tough time making the best choices. Start with the most obvious shopping trick: Don't shop hungry. Grocery shopping on an empty stomach is never a good idea because research has shown it inhibits your ability to make smart choices about what you wish to eat. A study published in *JAMA Internal Medicine* suggests that even short-term fasts can lead people to make more unhealthy food choices and put a higher quantity of high-calorie foods in their shopping carts. Shop after meals, not before, and bring a well-planned list! A *Journal of Nutrition Education and Behavior* study of more than 1,300 people discovered that shoppers who regularly wrote grocery lists also purchased healthier foods and had lower BMIs than those who didn't put pen to paper before heading to the store. Researchers hypothesize that shopping lists keep us organized, which in turn helps us fend off diet-derailing impulse buys. (See you later, candy aisle.) Before heading to the supermarket to stock up, spend a few minutes in your kitchen taking inventory, and then write a list. Organize it by category to prevent zigzagging all over the store, which increases the odds that you'll walk by a tempting packaged treat that'll end up in your cart.

Once you've crossed everything off your list, head to the self-checkout aisle. According to a study by IHL Consulting Group, impulse purchases dipped 32.1 percent for women and 16.7 percent for men when they scanned their own items and swiped their credit cards themselves. Did you know that 80 percent of candy and 61 percent of salty-snack purchases are unplanned? The impulse grab often happens when you are waiting in line flanked by single-serve chip bags and shelves filled with chocolate bars.

5. Order Right at Restaurants

We've all been there—you think you're going to pick something healthy off the menu until you get sidetracked by the special. Look up the restaurant menu before you go and decide on your order before you even walk in the door. You'll be less likely to order the smothered tater tots on impulse. When you go unprepared, consider a few tricks that can make restaurant meals a little healthier.

Start by noticing "health halos," the perception that everything from a healthy-seeming restaurant is a good pick. When people guess the number of calories in a sandwich coming from a "healthy" restaurant, they estimate that it has, on average, 35 percent fewer calories than it actually does, according to a study in the *Journal of Consumer Research*.

Think twice about "combo" and "value" meals, too. A study in the *Journal of Public Policy & Marketing* shows that compared to when they order à la carte, diners pick up a hundred or more extra calories by opting for the cheaper "value meals." When you order items bundled together, you might end up with more food than you need or want, which can lead to overeating. To keep your weight in check, order your food piecemeal instead.

At sit-down restaurants, a salad or soup appetizer can be a smart pick if it's the right kind. While some appetizers (think mozzarella sticks) add more calories to your meal, a series of studies from Penn State University found that biting into an apple or sipping a broth-based soup before eating dinner out can reduce your total calorie intake at the meal by as much as 20 percent.

Just remember to ask for sauces or dressing on the side. Though these emulsions add flavor to a dish, they're also frequently packed with added sugar and a whole host of other unhealthy stuff that makes shedding pounds that much harder. By asking for the sauce or dressing on the side, you have more control over how much of it you eat, and you could easily save yourself a few hundred calories. One sauce you should definitely ask for? Hot cayenne pepper sauce. Cayenne pepper contains capsaicin, an appetite suppressant; a study in *American Journal of Clinical Nutrition* found that people who ate capsaicin consumed 200 fewer calories at their next meal. A few dashes can help you cut back on calories, and researchers have also found that capsaicin can help you lose belly fat fast.

6. Get Chilly

Your environment can play a supporting role in your

weight-loss efforts. To start blasting away fat, turn down your heat (or crank the AC) before bed. A study published in the journal *Diabetes* found that participants who slept in bedrooms at a chilly 66 degrees burned almost twice as much fat after a few weeks as those who slept in rooms that were a neutral 75 or a toasty 81 degrees.

7. Hide the Sweet Stuff

Though you may think that strong willpower is a necessary factor in overcoming downtime grazing, experts say that your success is more dependent on your food environment than anything else. "If you happen to get bored and there is nothing but healthy food available in your house, you likely won't choose to eat it unless you're actually hungry," Jennifer Neily, MS, RDN, of Neily on Nutrition told us. Simply reorganizing your pantry staples could translate into serious calorie savings. A study published in the *Journal of Marketing* suggests that people are more likely to overeat small treats from a transparent package than from an opaque one. For this reason, many nutritionists suggest keeping indulgent foods in the pantry on a high shelf so that you're less apt to mindlessly grab them.

How Many Calories Do I Need?

Some people find counting calories as annoying as reading company-wide emails. Others really get into the game. No matter where you fall on this preference spectrum, simply estimating your total daily calories can help you become a more mindful eater. The chart here should make calorie estimating easier. It shows a rough estimate of your daily calorie needs if you want to maintain your weight. To lose weight, so the idea goes, you need to eat fewer calories. Of course, we all know that some foods/calories/energy affect your body/hunger/blood sugar differently than other foods do. The 150 calories in a can of soda is not the same as 150 calories of salmon and brussels sprouts, for example.

MALES			
Age	Sedentary	Moderately active	Active
18	2,400	2,800	3,200
19–20	2,600	2,800	3,000
21–25	2,400	2,800	3,000
26–30	2,400	2,600	3,000
31–35	2,400	2,600	3,000
36–40	2,400	2,600	2,800
41–45	2,200	2,600	2,800
46–50	2,200	2,400	2,800
51–55	2,200	2,400	2,800
56–60	2,200	2,400	2,600
61–65	2,000	2,400	2,600
66–70	2,000	2,200	2,600
71–75	2,000	2,200	2,600
76+	2,000	2,200	2,400

Age	Sedentary	Moderately active	Active
18	1,800	2,000	2,400
19–20	2,000	2,200	2,400
21–25	2,000	2,200	2,400
26–30	1,800	2,000	2,400
31–35	1,800	2,000	2,200
36–40	1,800	2,000	2,200
41–45	1,800	2,000	2,200
46–50	1,800	2,000	2,200
51–55	1,600	1,800	2,200
56–60	1,600	1,800	2,200
61–65	1,600	1,800	2,000
66–70	1,600	1,800	2,000
71–75	1,600	1,800	2,000
76+	1,600	1,800	2,000

Chapter 2 Action Summary

- Hop on a scale to determine your weight and then multiply that number by 0.05 to figure out the number of pounds you should lose in order to gain healthier heart benefits. Use that goal to keep you motivated as you embrace the lifestyle changes in our plan.

- Sweep your kitchen. Toss processed foods loaded with empty calories and added sugars. (We're talking about baked goods, chips, crackers, pretzels, soda, and such.)

- Practice mindful eating. Plan your meals. Slow down your scarfing. Be aware of the nutrition content of your meals.

- Break the habit of fast-food restaurant eating.

Pile Your Plate with Plants

Eat to your heart's (and arteries')
content with selections from this cornucopia
of delicious produce.

HAVE YOU TRIED LUCAMA? *What's that, you say? Oh, well, it's a Peruvian fruit that looks like a cross between a mango and a nashi pear. What's a nashi pear? Oh, well . . .*

Our point is, every other day there seems to be an exotic new plant food available to help you lose weight, supercharge your immune system, and make the grocery stores hit their revenue goals. Many of these trendy so-called superfoods are expensive—have you priced açai berries lately?—and hard to find (*moringa oleifera*, for instance) at the local Piggly Wiggly.

The truth is your heart doesn't need Tiger Nuts; the understated (and cheap) chickpea will do it just fine. When it comes to heart health, many common, easy-to-find foods deserve "super" status, from the boring stalk of broccoli to the humble peanut. Vegetables, fruits, and legumes are all super heart foods.

Study after study shows that people who eat the most produce and legumes have a lower risk of heart disease and other health problems, too. These foods are filled with fiber, vitamins, minerals, and other compounds that are good for you, such as antioxidants, which have become pretty famous for their preventive powers. In a study in the *European Journal of Epidemiology*, the women who ate the most foods rich in antioxidants had a 28 to 40 percent lower risk of a heart attack than those who ate less of these supercharged foods. The researchers suggest that antioxidants may have protective effects, and that some antioxidants might even work together to provide bonus benefits. So double and triple up!

If you think you can skip out on super heart foods and consume critical nutrients in supplement form instead, we have some lucama powder you may be interested in. A sweeping research review published in the *Journal of the American College of Cardiology* concluded that dietary supplements are *not* a proven way to reduce your risk of heart disease. Many nutrition experts contend that the best way to consume your nutrients is through whole, minimally processed foods, which have vitamins, minerals, and more already packaged inside by Mother Nature.

Your Healthy Heart Diet Goal: Eat at least four to six servings of vegetables, two to four servings of fruits, and a serving of legumes every day. Bonus points if you can do more, and if you can hit the mark of 10 servings of produce per day, consider yourself a bona fide nutritional superstar. It's not hard to do if you have the goods on hand.

TURN YOUR KITCHEN INTO A FARM STAND

In the 7-Day Healthy Heart Diet, we aim for four to six servings of vegetables every day, minimum. Minimum! That may sound like a lot, but it's not hard to hit that number. If you can fill your plate half full with vegetables at every meal, you're there.

"I try to figure out all the different ways I can sneak vegetables into a meal," says Judith Wylie-Rosett, EdD, RD, division head for health promotion and nutrition research at Albert Einstein College of Medicine. "We tend to think of eating salad *or* a vegetable. We tend to think of vegetables being separate from the entrée. You can put a lot of vegetables into entrées."

For example, let's say you're making macaroni and cheese for dinner tonight because your kids love it. Add some finely chopped cauliflower or broccoli to the mix, recommends Wylie-Rosett. Keep frozen vegetables on hand to make this sneakiness even easier. They are just as nutritious—sometimes even more nutritious—than the fresh ones.

"They're flash-frozen and you pop 'em in the microwave, as opposed to something that's been on the grocery store shelf for a while that may actually have been sprayed down with water to keep it looking fresher for several days," says Wylie-Rosett. It's faster than fast food! There are many ways to add frozen vegetables to your favorite meals. For example, steam frozen veggies and stir them into soup to make it heartier.

Any vegetable is probably better than no vegetable (unless you have some weird asparagus allergy or something). Veggies are packed with nutrients that can make you healthier, and you can even maximize those benefits by mixing things up. Go out on a limb and try something new.

"I recommend variety," says Erin Peisach, RDN, CLT, a San Diego–based dietician. "People can get stuck with their same three fruits and vegetables. I give clients a list so they can get inspired to find something new and find a recipe to incorporate it."

Don't be afraid to pick up something new based on what looks freshest at the farmer's market or grocery store. When you bring them home, store 'em where you can see 'em. You're more likely to grab fruits and veggies over less-healthy options if they're ready to eat and in plain sight. Katie Cavuto, MS, RD, the dietitian for the Philadelphia Phillies and Flyers, suggests keeping washed and prepared veggies like carrots, cucumbers, peppers, and sugar snap peas in the front of the fridge so they aren't overlooked. Apples, bananas, oranges, and pears fare well as sweet snacks and should be kept on the counter where everyone can see them.

After all, vegetables may be nutritional superstars, but

fruits deserve accolades, too. Fruits are sweet and delicious, and their sweetness is naturally occurring and comes with a side of fiber, antioxidants, vitamins and other helpful nutrients. Fiber is the big one. And you don't get it when you drink orange or apple juice. Fiber slows the absorption of fructose into your bloodstream so you don't get the wild blood sugar highs and lows that can trigger hunger.

When it comes to fruit, we want you to aim for two to four servings a day. Switch up the types of fruit you eat so you get different kinds of vitamins and minerals each day. The following vegetables and fruits are super heart foods, so work them into your diet as much as you can.

VEGETABLES

Acorn squash

Besides serving up a third of your day's fiber, a 1-cup serving of this dark-green squash, a highly nutritious, naturally sweet veggie, contains 30 percent of your daily vitamin C needs. The body uses the nutrient to form muscle and blood vessels, and it can even boost the fat-burning effects of exercise, according to Arizona State University researchers.

Asparagus

Your favorite grilled veggie is more than just a tasty side dish. Because asparagus is rich in folate—just four spears contain 89 micrograms of the nutrient, or roughly 22 percent of your recommended daily value—it's a super healthy carb for those living with diabetes. According to a meta-analysis published in *Diabetes Research and Clinical Practice*, folic acid can lower cardiovascular risk among patients with type 2 diabetes by reducing homocysteine levels, an amino acid that's been linked to increased risk of mortality in diabetic patients.

Beets

Beets contain a powerful nutrient called betaine, which lends the root veggie its rich red hue as well as fights inflammation, boosts metabolism, improves your mood, and turns off your fat genes. Beets also contain nitrate, which your body converts into nitric oxide, a gas that affects blood vessel expansion and contraction and may reduce blood pressure over time with regular intake.

Carrots

You probably know them for their vision-protecting reputation, but carrots have a lot more to offer. The (usually) orange vegetable reduces cholesterol and protects the heart, thanks to a plethora of vitamins and minerals. One study in the *Journal of Human Health and Hypertension* reported that eating raw carrots is linked with lower blood pressure, so pack some carrot sticks in your lunch or shred some into a salad.

Cherry Tomatoes

Americans eat more tomatoes and tomato products than any other non-starchy "vegetable." And tomatoes are a good choice because they are particularly rich in lycopene, an antioxidant that, unlike most nutrients in fresh produce, actually increases after cooking and processing. Dozens of studies suggest a relationship between regular intake of lycopene-rich tomatoes and a lower risk of cardiovascular disease, skin damage, and certain cancers. Since the disease-fighting polyphenols in tomatoes occur in the skin, grape and cherry tomatoes are ideal. Tomato sauces can also be a good choice if they're not packed with sugar and sodium—more on that in Chapter 6. We like Rao's Homemade Marinara Sauce, since it has simple ingredients (mostly just tomatoes, olive oil, and seasonings) and only 80 calories, 3 g sugar, and 340 mg sodium per ½-cup.

Cruciferous Vegetables

Rich sources of highly available calcium and iron, cruciferous vegetables like cabbage have the powerful ability to "turn off" inflammation markers that are thought to promote heart disease. In a study of more than 1,000 Chinese women, published in the *Journal of the Academy of Nutrition and Dietetics*, those who ate the most cruciferous vegetables (about 1.5 cups per day) had 13 percent less inflammation than those who ate the least. Credit a compound called sulforaphane in cruciferous vegetables. In addition to cabbage, the cruciferous family includes broccoli, cauliflower, and kale, and they're all heart-smart choices.

Jicama

This Central American root vegetable looks like a potato or turnip but is juicy and slightly sweet. One cup of jicama contains just 49 calories yet is loaded with 6 grams of fiber. Jicama also packs a hefty dose of vitamin C, which helps to reduce cholesterol oxidation, a dangerous process that makes cholesterol more likely to cause arterial damage. You can slice jicama and eat it raw or boil it like a potato until soft.

Leafy Greens

You've been told to eat them over and over again for good reason: spinach, swiss chard, and other dark green leafy veggies. These greens contain many beneficial nutrients, from vitamin K to fiber to folate—and more. There's one particular mineral in these superstars that's essential for your heart: magnesium. A lack of magnesium slows down energy metabolism, which can result in palpitations, insomnia, fatigue, headaches, and muscle cramps, and ultimately, high blood pressure, diabetes, and atherosclerosis, a cardiovascular disease.

Onions

They're worth the tears. Canadian researchers discovered that a type of gut-healthy insoluble fiber found in onions, called oligofructose, can increase levels of ghrelin—a hormone that controls hunger—and decrease blood sugar levels. Plus, thanks to their bioactive sulfur-containing compounds, onions can help lower cholesterol, ward off hardening of the arteries (arteriosclerosis), and help maintain healthy blood pressure, according to a study published in the *British Journal of Nutrition*. Pro tip: Sauté your onions for better benefits; the same study found the cholesterol-lowering properties were stronger in cooked onions than in those eaten raw.

Radishes

Eat red vegetables like radishes. Their red hue comes from anthocyanins, a group of phytochemical compounds that has been shown to burn fat and reduce inflammation, insulin resistance, and bad cholesterol. In a Japanese study, rats fed radishes for three weeks showed reduced levels of bad cholesterol and insulin and a bump in good cholesterol. Use radishes as a salad garnish or taco-topper, or eat them whole as a high-fiber, belly-filling snack.

Sweet potatoes

Like bananas, these orange root vegetables are rich in heart-protecting carotenoids. Sweet potatoes are also rich in vitamin B_6 and potassium, which are important for boosting heart health. Just don't corrupt them with sugar and marshmallows. Try our baked sweet potato fries recipe on page 182.

Is Wine a Super Heart Food?

We've all heard it a zillion times: Red wine is a healthy choice for your heart, since it contains the antioxidant resveratrol. But if you're citing that little piece of info as an excuse to drink half a bottle of cabernet every night, you are making a mistake. Wine is loaded with sugars and calories, and it goes straight into fat storage. In *The 7-Day Healthy Heart Diet*, we recommend doing without alcohol—not just for 7 days but for at least for 14. Your liver may welcome the break! Besides, 7 to 14 days of being a teetotaler will help you lose more weight and may break your habit of nightly nightcaps. "Most people don't know—or don't want to know—that wine and other alcoholic drinks are associated with breast cancer incidence, says registered dietician Christine M. Palumbo, MBA, RDN. "But it's a truth that shouldn't be ignored." And if you do drink, stick to just one.

FRUITS

Apples

Munching an apple each day can help prevent metabolic syndrome, a disorder associated with abdominal fat, cardiovascular disease, and diabetes. Red or green, any variety of apple is a low-calorie, nutrient-dense source of fiber, which research has proven to be integral to reducing visceral fat. A study at Wake Forest Baptist Medical Center found that for every 10-gram increase in soluble fiber eaten per day, visceral fat was reduced by 3.7 percent over five years.

Avocado

This fatty fruit provides a solid dose of monounsaturated and polyunsaturated fats that help lower LDL (bad cholesterol) as well as reducing your risk for cardiovascular disease and inflammation, Adam Splaver, MD, clinical cardiologist and cofounder of Nano Health Associates told us. Top your lunch with just one-quarter of the calorie-dense fruit to reap the benefits. Or enjoy this take on the millennial classic, avocado toast: Mash one-quarter or one-half of an avocado with a squeeze of lemon, a dash of hot sauce, and some salt and pepper before slathering it on your whole-wheat toast in the morning, and you'll easily stay full until lunchtime.

Bananas

These perfectly packaged fruits contain phytosterols, which are compounds that have LDL cholesterol-lowering effects, according to a study in the *Journal of Nutrition*. Bananas are also rich in three different types of carotenoids (provitamin A carotenoids, beta-carotene, and alpha-carotene) that the body converts into vitamin A. According to an article in the *Food and Nutrition Bulletin,* foods containing high levels of carotenoids have been shown to protect against chronic disease, including certain cancers, cardiovascular disease, and diabetes.

Berries

Next time you head out to the supermarket, don't forget to fill your cart with strawberries, blueberries, and raspberries. "Berries are rich in antioxidants, which help protect from free radical damage. These free radicals could potentially increase the risk of heart disease and cancer," Suzanne Fisher, registered dietitian, licensed nutritionist, and founder of Fisher Nutrition Systems told us. "Berries are also an excellent source of fiber and are low-glycemic, meaning they do not produce sugar spikes which could lead to insulin resistance."

Cherries

Sweeten up your meals and lower your blood pressure in one fell swoop by making cherries part of your diet today. Not only are cherries packed with fiber, quercetin, and vitamin C, but a study published in the February 2015 edition of *Clinical Nutrition* has linked their resveratrol content to significant reductions in systolic blood pressure, as well.

Grapefruit

Consider this your new favorite appetizer. A study in the journal *Metabolism* suggests that eating half a grapefruit before meals may help reduce visceral fat and lower cholesterol levels. Participants in the six-week study who ate grapefruit with every meal saw their waists shrink by up to an inch! Researchers attribute the effects to a combination of phytochemicals and the vitamin C in the grapefruit. What's more, a study review from the UK suggests that people who consume grapefruit on a regular basis decrease their systolic blood pressure by about 2.4 points on average. Grapefruit extracts might make blood vessels more flexible, the researchers say.

Grapes

These little orbs contain antioxidants such as resveratrol that can benefit your heart. Researchers in Italy found that people who ate grapes every day for three weeks had healthier blood-clotting activity. Study subjects ate 5 grams of grapes per kilogram of body weight. That's about 2 cups (two servings!) for a 130-pound person.

Kiwi

This fuzzy little fruit is rich in vitamin C and antioxidants. People who ate at least one kiwi a week had a reduced odds of insulin resistance and other markers of heart trouble, according to research from Spain.

24 Simple Tricks to Make Produce Last Longer

Have you ever stocked up your fridge with tons of healthy fruits and hearty veggies, only to watch them turn into a soggy soup of decomposed plant matter? It ain't pretty. And it's a waste of food and money. You'll end up eating more if you keep your produce fresh for as long as possible. Try these simple tips and tricks to do just that.

- Buy produce that is not bruised.
- Buy packaged produce that is refrigerated or surrounded by ice.
- Keep onions, potatoes, and tomatoes out of the fridge. Store these in a cool, dry area instead.
- Put unripe bananas on the counter. Then move them to the fridge once they ripen.
- Keep ethylene-emitting produce (avocados, kiwis, tomatoes, melons) away from ethylene-sensitive foods (apples, broccoli, carrots, lettuce). Keep bananas away from your other produce, since they produce high amounts of ethylene gas. Ethylene, a natural plant hormone, degrades plant cells, causing fruits and vegetables to ripen and get soft too quickly.
- Don't store produce near a gas stove or oven, and avoid storing produce near areas with smoke or heat.
- Keep tomatoes at room temperature and away from sunlight, and do not store them in plastic.
- Keep your fridge clean.
- Don't overstock your fridge.
- Store fresh fruits and vegetables in the fridge at a temperature of 40°F or below.
- Store fresh herbs and salad greens in the fridge in tightly sealed bags filled with a small amount of air.
- Store citrus fruits in the fridge in a mesh or perforated plastic bag.

- Wrap celery in aluminum foil before storing it in the veggie bin of the fridge.
- Stow broccoli, carrots, and lettuce separately in dry bags in your fridge's crisper.
- To store pineapples, cut the leafy top off and place in fridge upside down.
- Refrigerate all produce that is purchased pre-cut or packaged.
- Chop dried onions and chives and store them in an empty water bottle in the freezer.
- Store chopped salad greens in the fridge in a bowl lined with paper towels and cover with plastic wrap.
- Store roots such as ginger and turmeric in the freezer.
- Keep meats and fruits in separate areas of the fridge to avoid contamination.
- Store mushrooms in a brown paper bag in the fridge or another cool, dry area.
- Moisture causes mold, so do not wash berries until you're ready to eat them.
- Don't cut produce until you absolutely have to.
- Spritz lemon juice on cut apples, avocados, and guacamole to keep them from browning.

LEGUMES

The next group of super heart foods is one that is highly underrated: legumes, a selection that includes beans, peas, chickpeas, lentils, and soybeans.

One of the superstar nutrients in legumes is resistant starch, a type of carbohydrate that passes through your gut undigested. Resistant starch feeds your healthy gut bacteria, which in turn produces a fatty acid called butyrate that encourages more efficient fat oxidation. Higher levels of butyrate reduce inflammation in your body and help reduce insulin resistance, as well.

Promoting insulin sensitivity, as legumes do, is a critical factor in reducing your odds of diabetes. For example, as you digest legumes, they increase production of proteins involved in sugar metabolism. High in fiber, beans and other legumes are famous for their ability to help people reduce blood cholesterol levels.

"In general, people don't tend to eat enough legumes," says registered dietitian and recipe developer Peisach. "There are so many great recipes using them, and they are high in fiber, proteins, and minerals—and they're cheap."

It's easy to add legumes to soups and salads, burritos, and quesadillas, and so much more. Aim for a daily serving (about ½-cup), and try these:

Black beans

A half cup of black beans not only packs 3.1 grams of resistant starch, but it also carries nearly 20 grams of protein and 14 grams of filling fiber, making black beans a delicious fat-fighting triple threat. Plus, black beans are high in anthocyanins, antioxidants associated with lowering inflammation. According to a study in the journal *Nutrients*, when patients with metabolic syndrome consumed a meal with black beans, their levels of insulin measured right after a meal were lower than in subjects who ate a meal with a similar amount of fiber or a similar amount of antioxidants. High levels of postprandial glucose and insulin have been implicated in increases in inflammation and oxidative stress—making black beans a potent Western-diet inflammation-fighter.

Chickpeas

People who regularly eat chickpeas and hummus made from chickpeas tend to have a higher intake of heart-healthy nutrients, including fiber, magnesium, potassium, and more, according to a study published in *Journal of Nutrition & Food Sciences*. Chickpea eaters were also 51 percent less likely to have elevated blood sugar levels than the people who skipped garbanzos. Pop these little legumes on a salad, or make hummus with our recipe (on page 194), which only requires seven ingredients: chickpeas, garlic, cumin, lemon juice, salt, tahini, and olive oil. If you're using dried chickpeas, soak them in water overnight so that they soften and lend your hummus an ultra-velvety texture.

Edamame

Soybean pods, which are often labeled as "edamame" at grocery stores and restaurants, are a great anytime snack because they're an excellent source of magnesium, folate, and potassium. These nutrients can help lower blood pressure and support heart health, reducing your risk for heart disease. Plus, the fiber in edamame may protect the heart by boosting the body's ability to produce low-density lipoprotein (LDL) receptors, which act like bouncers, pulling that "bad" cholesterol out of the blood. Nosh on dry-roasted edamame, or heat up frozen pods for a satisfying snack. Tofu is a good form of soy, too!

Kidney beans

You know that beans are a great source of fiber, but you may not realize the extent to which kidney beans meet this expectation. In fact, these red beans provide a whopping 14 grams—that's the same as in more than three servings of oatmeal! For that reason, these pulses can be considered an effective blood-sugar control pill, as their unique resistant-starch fibers take longer to digest, making them a very "low glycemic" carbohydrate that helps prevent blood sugar spikes. A recent study found diabetics who ate one cup of beans every day for 3 months saw better improvements in fasting blood sugar, cholesterol, and even body weight than a group who ate 1 cup of equally fibrous, whole-wheat products.

Lentils

Lentils have been a part of the human diet for some 13,000 years for a reason. They're packed with protein and fiber, and are touted by health experts for their ability to reduce inflammation, lower cholesterol, promote fat metabolism, and dampen appetites. Lentils are a resistant starch, a slow-digesting fiber that triggers the release of acetate—a molecule in the gut that tells the brain when to stop eating. In fact, a systematic review of clinical trials found that people who ate a daily serving of lentils (about 3/4 cup) felt an average 31 percent fuller compared to a control diet. And a second study found a diet rich in blood-sugar-stabilizing foods like lentils could reduce disease-related inflammation by 22 percent.

ADD HIGH-NUTRIENT FLAVOR ENHANCERS

A little flavor can go a long way toward promoting heart health, if you choose the right ones. Stock up on these:

Chocolate

Great news, chocoholics: Dozens of studies show that people who consume cocoa—as a hot drink or eaten as dark chocolate—are in much better cardiovascular shape than those who don't. One 9-year study in the journal *Circulation Heart Failure* found women who ate one to two servings of high-quality chocolate per week had a 32 percent lower risk of developing heart failure than those who said no to the cocoa. And a second long-term study found that men who ate the most chocolate–about one-third of a cup of dark chocolate chips per week–had a 17 percent reduced risk of stroke compared to those who didn't consume chocolate. Researchers attribute cocoa's health benefits to polyphenols and flavonols, anti-inflammatory compounds that help protect the heart. But these people weren't downing Milky Way bars. Opt for dark chocolate that's at least 70 percent cacao to reap the maximum antioxidant benefits. We love Endangered Species Dark Chocolate and Dove Dark Chocolate Squares.

Cinnamon

This warming spice helps control blood sugar. One study found that adding a heaping teaspoon of cinnamon to a starchy meal is as effective as older generation diabetes drugs at stabilizing blood sugar and warding off insulin spikes. And a second study in the *Journal of Nutrition* found that when a meal contained a spice blend including cinnamon, antioxidant activity in the blood was increased by 13 percent and insulin response decreased by about 20 percent. Researchers theorize that cinnamaldehyde, cinnamon's active ingredient, works as a blood-sugar balancer by stimulating insulin receptors on cells and allowing excess sugar to move out of the blood. *Cassia* cinnamon is the variety you're most likely to find at the grocery store, but it's *Ceylon* cinnamon, a milder, pricier variety, that's touted by health experts. You can find true cinnamon online or in Indian marketplaces and spice shops.

Ginger

Ginger is more than the popular spice that livens up smoothies and sushi; this potent root can help your cholesterol levels, too. Ginger has been found to help reduce total cholesterol, LDL, and very low-density lipoprotein (VLDL) levels, the most dangerous kind, when subjects consumed three doses of 3-gram ginger capsules. Researchers attribute ginger's health benefits to *gingerols*, compounds that are antioxidant, anti-inflammatory, and antibacterial. Grate some fresh ginger into your next smoothie or tea for some heart-boosting benefits.

Rosemary

It's not just a staple when you're marinating your lemon chicken; this flavorful herb is also a powerful anti-inflammatory, thanks to its high concentration of antioxidant compounds. (In fact, you'll often see "rosemary extract" listed on your natural processed goods as an antioxidant natural preservative.) Scientists believe the anti-inflammatory activity comes from the presence of carnosic acid and carnosol, two polyphenolic compounds in rosemary and found in a study published in the journal *BMC Complementary and Alternative Medicine* to effectively inhibit the production of pro-inflammatory cytokines.

Tea

Steep a cup. Teas—black, green, and white—are loaded with antioxidants that'll benefit your heart. In a recent study published in the *American Journal of Medicine*, people who regularly drank 1 cup or more of tea per day had a reduced risk of cardiovascular events compared to those who sipped less. And in another study in *Nutrition Research*, every 3.4 ounces of tea consumed daily was linked to a 0.6-point drop in systolic blood pressure.

Dress Salads Properly

To hit your daily vegetable count, you'll probably eat some salads here and there. If you dress your salads with a squeeze of lemon and some pepper in an attempt to save calories, you may miss out on some of the vital vitamins in your bowl. According to Iowa and Ohio State University researchers, pairing a little bit of fat with your veggies helps the body absorb their cancer-fighting and heart-healthy nutrients, such as lycopene and beta-carotene. Make your own dressings with our recipes on page 196, or pick one at the store that contains less than 250 milligrams of salt and less than 3 grams of sugar per 2 tablespoons. These are a few of our favorites.

Eat This! Annie's Organic Caesar Dressing

Per 2 Tbsp: 110 calories, 11 g fat (1 g saturated fat), 240 mg sodium, 3 g carbs (2 g sugars, 0 g fiber), 1 g protein

If you're yearning for an indulgent flavor factor to keep your salad streak going, Annie's organic Caesar trumps most commercial brands; many inject their formulas with belly-ballooning fat and salt. Plus, this Caesar is egg-free and non-GMO.

Eat This! Annie's Organic
Red Wine & Olive Oil Vinaigrette

Per 2 Tbsp: 140 calories, 15 g fat (2 g saturated fat), 190 mg sodium, 0 g carbs, 0 g protein

Annie's adds tang and body to your salads without breaking your calorie budget. Two tablespoons pack in less than 150 calories and boast 15 grams of fat coming from extra-virgin olive oil. EVOO is brimming with oleic acid, a monounsaturated fat that has been shown to prevent heart disease.

Eat This! Bragg Vinaigrette

Per 2 Tbsp: 90 calories, 9 g fat (1.5 g saturated fat), 60 mg sodium, 3 g carbs (2 g sugars, 0 g fiber), 0 g protein

Apple cider vinegar, which has been linked to weight loss and appetite suppression, is the top ingredient in Bragg's healthful vinaigrette. It's sweetened with a drop of organic honey and liquid aminos, and it's balanced with a dash of black pepper for a low-sodium sauce that's as wholesome as it tastes.

Eat This! Hilary's Ranch Chia

Per 2 Tbsp: 35 calories, 3 g fat (2.5 g saturated fat), 150 mg sodium, 2 g carbs (1 g sugars, 0 g fiber,), 0 g protein

Instead of relying on a fatty base of vegetable oil and buttermilk, Hilary's concocts its creamy ranch with hearty coconut milk. To add to the benefits, this dressing packs in heart-healthy chia seeds, which load each bite with a dose of omega-3s.

Eat This! Organic Girl Avocado Cilantro

Per 2 Tbsp: 120 calories, 13 g fat (1.5 g saturated fat), 80 mg sodium, 2 g carbs, (1 g sugars, 0 g fiber), 0 g protein

If the avocado on your countertop isn't yet ripe for use, don't fret—you can still get the coveted creamy flavor with this organic offering. Organic Girl boasts a kick of jalapeños and invigorating lime juice as well as satiating unsaturated fats that help you absorb many veggies' fat-soluble nutrients. Squirt this over a Mexican-style salad when you're short on time to make fresh guac.

Eat This! Primal Kitchen Lemon Turmeric Vinaigrette & Marinade

Per 2 Tbsp: 90 calories, 10 g fat (1.5 g saturated fat), 95 mg sodium, 1 g carbs (1 g sugar, 0 g fiber), 0 g protein

Curcumin, the main antioxidant in turmeric, has been shown to fight inflammation—a key driver of weight gain. After you've drizzled your greens with the golden stuff, add a dash of black pepper. The zesty spice helps increase turmeric's bioavailability.

Eat This! **Tessemae's Green Goddess**

Per 1 Tbsp: 80 calories, 9 g fat (1.5 g saturated fat), 90 mg sodium, 0 g carbs, 0 g protein

Unlike our other contenders, Tessemae's serving size is trimmed down to a mere tablespoon. However, even if you double it to two, the nutritionals bennies remain quite impressive. Instead of stuffing in deleterious amounts of sodium and sugar, Tessemae's flavors its sauce with organic tamari, EVOO, and turmeric.

Chapter 3 Action Summary

- Turn your kitchen into a farm stand: Keep a variety of vegetables and fruits on hand.

- Tap the power of resistant starches. Bean up.

- Boost the nutritional profiles of meals with flavor enhancers.

4

Exercise Your Heart Every Day

Make your diet work harder with all the right moves.

THINK OF YOUR HEART-HEALTHY diet as Batman. Exercise is Robin. They work much better together than apart, and if your heart is Gotham City, you need both of these superheroes on your team.

That's why we've developed an exercise plan as part of the 7-Day Healthy Heart Diet. If your goal is weight loss, changing your diet to reduce carbs and calories is the most effective strategy. Exercise won't do nearly as much. In fact, exercise can trigger hunger and undermine weight loss if you're not careful. However, if heart health is your goal, exercising your body is equally important as feeding your body the right fuel. Together, a heart-healthy diet and exercise have a synergistic relationship, according to a recent study conducted in Spain. For ten years, researchers there monitored people who closely followed the heart-healthy Mediterranean diet but did no exercise, people exercised but did not diet, and people who both exercised regularly and ate heart-healthy foods. While all the participants lowered their risk of cardiovascular disease (CVD) somewhat, only those who both exercised and ate healthfully slashed their CVD risk by 75 percent!

Exercise is essential for heart health for many reasons. It trains your heart, a giant muscle, to pump more efficiently. It burns off cholesterol and other artery-clogging fats. It keeps your arteries flexible, reducing the odds that they will narrow and clog. It curbs inflammation that would otherwise harm your heart and arteries over time. And it helps you lose weight so your heart doesn't have to work so hard 24/7.

Even for people with a genetic susceptibility to cardiovascular disease, exercise is a powerful shield, suggests research from Stanford University. A study there found that people who had the highest grip strengths, levels of physical activity, and fitness levels had reduced risks of coronary heart disease and atrial fibrillation, a heart rhythm abnormality that can literally make your heart stop dead. The benefits of exercise were especially pronounced in the study participants with high genetic risk for these heart problems. They had a 49 percent reduced risk of coronary heart disease and a 60 percent reduced risk of atrial fibrillation.

Unfortunately, as you might guess, many Americans fall short when it comes to being physically active. Only about

Forget Fruit Juice

While you might not think there's a huge difference between eating a whole piece of fruit and drinking fruit juice, nutritionally speaking, the two entities are most definitely not one and the same. Whereas whole fruit contains naturally occurring sugars and fiber that can help counteract the bad effects of too much sweet stuff, fruit juice is often loaded with added sugar (such as high-fructose corn syrup) and no fiber to speak of. According to a study led by Harvard School of Public Health researchers, eating more whole fruits, particularly blueberries, grapes, and apples, was significantly associated with a lower risk of type 2 diabetes. On the other hand, a greater consumption of fruit juices was associated with a higher risk of type 2 diabetes.

22 percent of American adults meet the government's Physical Activity Guidelines for Americans for aerobic and muscle-strengthening activity, according to the Centers for Disease Control and Prevention. The American Heart Association even issued a statement in 2016 urging Americans to sit less and move more. Study after study has found a simple fitness formula for a healthy heart: Get 150 minutes of moderate to vigorous exercise per week. We'll show you how to make hitting that minimum quota easy, and then we'll take your fitness level up a notch or two with a heart-healthy plan of interval and strength training.

Your Healthy Heart Diet Goal: Exercise 5 days a week. Our plan features 3 days of interval training, 2 days of strength training, and 2 rest days. You'll also be challenged to move more each day in between workouts, especially if you are sedentary or have a desk job.

Time Your Ticker

For a quick check of your heart's efficiency, check your resting heart rate. This is one of the easiest ways to monitor how well your heart pumps blood—especially if you have a fitness tracker or smartwatch. Your heart rate is simply the number of times your heart beats per minute. For the most telling marker, you want to assess your resting heart rate— the beat count when you are just chilling out. It should be much lower at rest than it is after, say, you've run around your block or have just done 30 burpees. Check it: Sit or lie down and just rest for 10 to 15 minutes, and then check the reading on your heart-rate monitor. Or do the low-tech pulse method: Take two fingers and rest them inside your wrist until you can feel the beat. Use a watch with a second hand and count the number of beats for 30 seconds, and then double it to get your magic number.

A normal resting heart rate is typically between 60 to 100 beats per minute. People who are very fit tend to be near the bottom of that range, and if you work out regularly, your heart may become more efficient at pumping, and your resting heart rate may decrease. Lower is better: Researchers in Norway and the UK found that for every 10 beats per minute increase in resting heart rate, risk of sudden cardiac death increased by 18 percent.

This chapter features a workout plan to help you build muscle, burn fat, and improve your cardiovascular health. It includes aerobic exercise, which is especially good at making your heart pump more efficiently. By checking your resting heart rate occasionally as you get fitter, you should notice a lower number over time. The workout also includes a strength training component. Training with weights or exercise bands or using your body weight is especially helpful for improving your blood sugar control, a key step in protecting your heart. This training can help you improve your body composition so that you have less fat and more muscle, a shift that is good for your heart.

THE HEALTHY HEART DIET FITNESS PLAN

Here's what we want you to do: First, sit less, walk more. You've heard about shooting for a goal of 10,000 steps a day for body-changing fitness? If you want to use a pedometer or smartphone app to track your steps, go right ahead. We find that annoyingly tedious. But there's no doubt that you'll do your heart a favor by reducing your butt-in-chair time. Sedentary days do not a healthy heart make. You've gotta move.

There are a lot of tricks for encouraging your body to do that every day. Just being mindful of opportunities to stand and walk will help. Here's a short list. You've no doubt heard some of these, but have you done them?

1) Take the stairs instead of the elevator.

2) Use the lavatory farthest from your office whenever you have to go at work.

3) Stand up whenever you talk on the phone.

4) Park in the farthest spot away from the door at work, at the mall, wherever.

5) Sign up for a charity walk.

6) Get a dog.

7) Buy an old-fashioned push mower and use it.

8) Zumba? No? OK, how 'bout polka?

9) Walk to pick up a gallon of milk instead of driving.

10) Conduct walking meetings at work.

11) March in place during TV commercials.

12) Set hourly walking reminders on your computer.

13) Never use the drive-thru.

14) Get off the bus one or two stops early on pleasant days.

15) Do ten squats while you brush your teeth.

16) Walk over to a colleague's office instead of calling or emailing.

17) Take a stroll after dinner.

18) Buy a new pair of running shoes.

19) Keep your telephone or cellphone upstairs.

20) Vacuum the rug; it needs it.

OK, we're moving more. Good. Now let's build some formal exercise into our week. By formal, we mean scheduled. If you create a workout "to-do" list and block out time for exercise, you'll be more likely to stick with it. Put your exercise time in your Outlook calendar as if it were an essential business meeting. Make it a habit, and soon you'll never want to miss a workout.

At the same time, tell others about your exercise plan. In a study of 100 middle-aged and older adults, researchers found that having social support was associated with strong adherence to a 12-month, at-home exercise program. Better yet, invite others to join you in your workout. A recent *JAMA Internal Medicine* study of nearly 4,000 couples found that people are more likely to stick to healthy habits when they team up with a partner. Think about it: Exercising with friends is more fun, and you'll be less likely to skip a session if a buddy is waiting for you.

For the 7-Day Healthy Heart Diet plan, we want you to mix 3 days of aerobic interval training with 2 days of strength or resistance training. With our schedule and your initiative to move more daily, you'll have no trouble nailing the 150 minutes of exercise recommended for good heart health. More likely, you'll log much more, at least 30 minutes a day, without allowing exercise to become a time burden.

Moderate aerobic activity like brisk walking, mowing the lawn, doing housework, and leisurely bike riding is good, but we'll encourage you to kick it up a notch. We'd like to see you do a mix of moderate and vigorous aerobic exercise, so we're advocating interval training 3 days a week. As you'll see in the workout below, intervals are nothing more than alternating between short bursts of faster, more intense exercise and longer, slower recovery segments.

You'll also do strength-training exercises to build all your major muscle groups at least twice a week. We want you to build muscle (don't worry, you won't become muscle-bound) because a stronger body moves and reacts more quickly, burns more calories, and more readily metabolizes blood sugar—all good for the heart. Strength training can be done with weights, weight machines, exercise bands, or even your own body weight. The important thing to accomplish is straining your muscle tissue in a controlled way so as to create micro-tears that encourage new muscle growth during recovery and repair. Even if you have never strength-trained before, you'll find our workout easy to learn and, we hope, fun.

On the following page, you'll find a sample workout schedule that shows you how to incorporate sessions into the week that follows your initial 7-day plan. After all, you're not going to stop exercising after one week. The key is to get three aerobic and two strength sessions and 2 rest days into each week.

The Schedule

1) **Monday:** Intervals
2) **Tuesday:** Strength
3) **Wednesday:** Rest
4) **Thursday:** Intervals
5) **Friday:** Strength
6) **Saturday:** Rest
7) **Sunday:** Intervals
8) **Monday:** Strength
9) **Tuesday:** Rest
10) **Wednesday:** Intervals
11) **Thursday:** Strength
12) **Friday:** Rest
13) **Saturday:** Intervals
14) **Sunday:** Strength

How to do it: Aerobic Intervals

Studies suggest that interval training, which alternates between intervals of high-intensity aerobic exercise and periods of lighter movement, can boost blood vessel function, improve fitness, and provide other benefits in less time than other training methods. That means you get more exercise benefits for less time actually spent exercising.

Researchers in Canada, for example, recently showed that men who did high-intensity interval training 3 times a week boosted their cardiovascular fitness as well as their blood sugar control. In a study from Denmark, women who did three interval training sessions a week reduced their body weight, waist circumference, and fat mass while increasing their muscle mass. What's more, they reduced their diastolic blood pressure and resting heart rate and improved their cholesterol levels and insulin concentration, a marker of blood sugar function.

Don't let the "high-intensity" part of interval training intimidate you—even beginners can do it, says Martin Gibala, PhD, a professor of kinesiology at McMaster University.

"A lot of people think that interval training is only about going as hard as you can go," says Gibala. The truth is that you can do interval training at a variety of paces. What's important is that you challenge yourself and keep getting better. "Just get out of your comfort zone," says Gibala. Try this:

33-Minute Interval Workout

3-minute warm-up: Walking or light jogging

4 minutes: Fast walking or running

3 minutes: Moderate walking or running

4 minutes: Fast walking or running

3 minutes: Moderate walking or running

4 minutes: Fast walking or running

3 minutes: Moderate walking or running

4 minutes: Fast walking or running

3 minutes: Moderate walking or running

2-minute cooldown: Walking or light jogging

The trick question, of course, is how fast is the fast part? Think about your exertion on a scale of 0 to 10, Gibala says. Zero is complete rest, and 10 is the pace at which you would sprint to save your child from being hit by a car. You can start with walking intervals where your fast walk is a 3, your moderate one, a 2. You can do sprint intervals where you run at an 8 and then go down to a 4. As your fitness increases, you will start moving faster and it will start to feel easier. In one week, your level 4 will be faster than it is today.

"The standard advice to check with your doctor before starting is sensible," he says. If you have certain conditions, you may need a modified workout plan. But he also notes that in most cases, "the greater risk to your health is just remaining sedentary." (One notable exception: people who do a lot of physical activity on the job. In a new study published in the journal *Heart*, men who exerted themselves at work actually had an increased risk of cardiovascular disease, and in their case, playing sports in their spare time did not reduce that risk. If you do physical labor, it's especially important to talk with your doctor before taking on any new exercise.)

You don't need a lot of time to build fitness and burn fat with interval training. Gibala recommends "exercise snacking," fitting in bits of exercise wherever you can. "Reframe your notion of exercise," he says. "It doesn't mean just changing into Spandex and going to a gym." His advice: "Sprinkle intervals into your life and do what works for you," says Gibala.

For example, when you take a walk, pick up the pace for a few seconds before resuming your normal clip. Step off the elevator a few floors early and walk the rest of the way. "Taking the stairs a few times a day can be a form of interval training," says Gibala. If you're standing in your office, do ten squats to increase your heart rate and activate those leg muscles. And if you like the interval pace shown above in the 33-minute session, but you don't have a half hour to spare, break it up into three 10-minute interval sessions. Make it fit your schedule, and you'll never skip a workout.

How to Do It: Strength Training

While aerobic exercise is critical, strength training is also an important part of a healthy routine. Researchers from the National Institutes of Health and Harvard University recently tracked 35,754 women's exercise habits for an average of nearly eleven years. They found that the women who lifted weights and did at least 120 minutes of aerobic exercise a week had the lowest risks of both cardiovascular disease and type 2 diabetes. Strength training has multiple benefits that could help your heart, the researchers noted. For example, it helps you increase your muscle mass, reduce your body mass index (BMI), and improve insulin sensitivity, contributing to better blood sugar control.

We're not asking you to become a bodybuilder. In fact, lifting very heavy weights could actually have a negative effect on your heart, says J. Derek Kingsley, PhD, an associate professor of health sciences at Kent State University. During these hard lifts, some people try to exhale forcefully with a closed windpipe, which is known as the Valsalva maneuver. (You may also do this when you strain in the bathroom.) This maneuver can raise blood pressure and might be hard on your blood vessels.

We won't ask you to test the limits of your strength, but we will help you boost it. This two-day-a-week whole-body circuit is designed for muscle building and fat loss.

The only equipment you'll need is a pair of dumbbells. Pick up weights that will challenge you without threatening an injury. Here's how to find the sweet spot: If you can do the move easily twelve times, you need a heavier dumbbell. If you can't make it past rep 8, grab a lighter one. Don't obsess about the number on the dumbbell. Form and technique are more important than poundage, says Kingsley, so think about how you use your body during each lift. For example, during bicep curls, stand against a wall to ensure that you aren't swinging to eke out the last few reps.

There's a simple way to assess how you are doing. "Are you doing more today than you did yesterday?" asks Kingsley. "That's how you make progress." Exercise is a lifelong endeavor, he says, and there's no better time than now to get started.

The Healthy Heart Strength Workout

Grab a set of dumbbells and do 8 to 10 repetitions of the following exercises. Repeat each exercise three times (3 sets) before moving on to the next exercise. Rest for one minute to 90 seconds between sets.

1) Chest Press
Grab a dumbbell in each hand. Lie on your back on a flat bench with your feet on the floor. Keep your back flat on the bench. Press the dumbbells up over your head with your elbows extended. Slowly lower them toward your chest and gently touch your chest. Press up again. This is 1 rep.

2) Front Squat
Stand with your feet about hip-width apart, turned a bit outward, with your weight on your heels. Hold a dumbbell

in each hand and rest them in front of your shoulders. With your back flat, lower your hips and bend your knees softly until your thighs are almost parallel with the floor. Rise to the starting position. This is 1 rep.

3) Lunge

Grab a dumbbell in each hand and stand with your feet about hip-width apart and your arms straight at your sides. With your back straight, step forward with one leg and lower the opposite knee toward the floor. Stand up to the starting position and repeat on the other side. This is 1 rep.

4) Front Raise

Stand with your feet slightly wider than your hips. Hold your dumbbells in front of your thighs with your arms extended. Slowly raise the dumbbells in front of you and slowly turn your arms so that your thumbs point upward by the time the dumbbells reach your shoulders. Lower back to the starting position. This is 1 rep.

5) Goblet Squat

Give your hips, butt, and legs—some of the biggest muscles in your body and major fat burners—extra attention with this second round of squats. Stand with your feet about shoulder width apart. Hold one dumbbell vertically with both hands in front of your chest. Keep your back straight and lightly press your elbows in toward your ribs as you lower your body. When your hips are below your knees, rise back to standing.

6) Lateral Lunge

Stand with your feet hip-width apart. With one dumbbell in

each hand, allow your arms to fully extend with the weights resting in front of your thighs. Take a wide step to the right side, keeping your feet parallel, and bend your right knee. Allow the weights to hang in front of you. Then bring your body back to the center and repeat on the other side. This is 1 rep.

7) Triceps Extension
Stand with one foot slightly in front of the other. Hold one dumbbell with both hands and press it up over your head. Bend your elbows and slowly lower the dumbbell behind your head until your elbows are at 90 degrees. This is 1 rep.

8) Hammer Curl
Stand with one foot slightly in front of the other and hold the dumbbells next to your thighs with your arms straight. Bend your elbows and slowly raise the dumbbells up to shoulder height. This is 1 rep.

You'll notice that our exercise plan includes rest days, and that's no mistake. Rest is important because your muscles need time to repair and rebuild after challenging workouts. When you don't give yourself enough time to relax between strength sessions, your body starts pumping out cortisol, a stress hormone that boosts fat storage and appetite—a killer combination for anyone looking to lose weight and burn fat. However, you don't have to spend rest days on the couch. Many athletes use rest days for *deloading*, a term that describes doing light exercise and stretches that promote flexibility and strength without compromising recovery, says Kingsley.

Tai chi and yoga are two great choices for deloading

on rest days because they keep your body moving while calming your mind, doubly benefitting your heart! In a study from Hong Kong, the people who practiced tai chi regularly for 9 months reduced their blood pressure, fasting blood sugar, and HbA1c by even more than the people who took up a brisk walking routine. Researchers in India found that people who did yoga every day reduced their fasting blood sugar, cholesterol levels, and triglycerides. Many fitness centers and local hospitals offer weekly classes in tai chi and yoga, and they're definitely worth a try.

Fit Tip

Set out your sneakers before you go to bed. Leaving your sneakers out within view of your bed will make it easier to get out of bed and remind you of why you're waking up early in the first place. Even better, set out your entire workout ensemble to cut down on the time it takes to get ready so you can get moving before you have time to change your mind.

OTHER WAYS TO BURN MORE CALORIES

One of the easiest ways to burn some extra calories is to get up from your chair at work; standing burns 50 more calories per hour than sitting, according to a British study. Use a standing desk at work or make your own by stacking books or boxes on your desk and standing up to work. At the very least, make sure you're taking a break every hour to stand up and stretch, and possibly go for a walk around the office.

(Set up a reminder on your phone or workplace calendar.)

Next, start chipping away at whatever household cleaning project you've been procrastinating on. Organize the tools in your garage. Go through all the clothes piled in the corner of your closet. Deep-clean something you've neglected. Keeping the house clean and the car sparkling in the driveway can be great sources of pride (and keep your mother from lecturing you during family visits), but doing so also forces you to move around. "Keep those arms moving while washing your car or scrubbing that oven," Jim White, RD, ACSM HFS, owner of Jim White Fitness and Nutrition Studios, told us. Squatting to reach low corners and stretching to get higher ones recruits different muscles in the body to get the job done. Not to mention, it forces you to move a lot more than if you were sitting on the couch ignoring your chores.

While you're at it, how's your garden looking? Of all the activities you can do in an effort to shed a few pounds, gardening is one of the most beneficial and relaxing options. A study from the University of Utah shows that people who garden are about 11 to 16 pounds lighter than those who don't! Bonus: In a pilot study from South Korea, older women who gardened twice a week for 15 sessions reduced their blood pressure, increased their HDL cholesterol levels, and had other beneficial increases in health markers. Put on some gardening gloves and get to planting.

If housework isn't your jam, then give your Amazon account a rest and go out shopping. "Constant walking around, standing in line, and bending to pick up that shirt you accidentally dropped all burns extra calories," White told us. There's no physical difference between walking on the treadmill and logging those steps in the mall—your body is going through the same motion. However, shopping fits more seamlessly into your day—and hey, you'll probably knock quite a few tasks off your to-do list with the extra motivation to move. Even better, lugging around those shopping bags will make your arms work even harder, contributing to greater overall exertion.

One more thing: Keep moving, and don't give up! If one of your kids comes down with the flu or something else happens that totally derails one of your workouts, just pick things back up as soon you can. A recent study published in *JAMA Internal Medicine* suggests that people who exercise regularly reduce their risk of dying of cardiovascular disease compared to inactive people, even if they fall short of the recommended guidelines. In other words, even if you don't follow our exercise plan 100 percent perfectly, you'll be way better off following it imperfectly than you would be if you didn't upgrade your exercise habits at all.

Build Movement into Your Day

For those days when you just can't squeeze in a formal exercise session, build opportunities to knock out a few bodyweight exercises into daily activities and tasks. Try these.

While You Watch TV
Per commercial break:
- A 20-second plank
- 10 jumping jacks
- 10 crunches
- 10 hip raises

According to a study conducted by the media agency Nielsen, there are a little more than 14 minutes of commercials played per television hour, just enough time to get in a quick workout during each break. Every time a commercial break pops on the screen, try doing a set of 10 of each exercise to keep your blood pumping and your muscles moving as you watch your favorite TV shows.

When You Open the Fridge

- 15 prisoner squats
- 20 alternating lunges

Do 15 high-intensity prisoner squats, which involves squatting as low as you can without letting your heels come off the ground, and then 20 alternating lunges (10 on each leg).

While You Use the Restroom

- 15 jump squats
- A 30-second wall sit

Add some quick workouts to each trip you make to the bathroom! Try doing 15 jump squats to tone your calves, thighs, and glutes before you head out of the bathroom. If you're in a public bathroom and don't want to draw attention to yourself, then do a 30-second wall sit against the door to strengthen your legs and core.

While You're Brushing Your Teeth

- 20 bodyweight squats

Even subconscious tasks like brushing your teeth can be a great time to exercise. Instead of mindlessly staring at the mirror, try incorporating some squats to get your muscles moving in the morning.

While You're Making Coffee

- 1 minute of marches with arm lifts
- 20 seated Russian twists
- 2 sets of 1-minute side elbow planks with twists (minute per side)

These exercises can easily be done while waiting for your morning coffee to brew. Takes just 5 minutes.

While You're Cooking

- 30 alternating lateral leg lifts
- 50 calf raises
- 20 counter push-ups

Work your legs out with 30 lateral leg lifts (15 per leg total) and 50 calf raises, which is basically just standing straight and going up onto your toes then slowly lowering back down. Then try some counter push-ups, which are exactly as they sound: using your countertop as a base for vertical push-ups.

When You're About to Go to Bed

- 1-minute forearm plank
- 20 seconds Tree Pose
- 20 seconds Warrior 3
- 20 seconds Downward Dog

End your day the right way and try to get some calming exercise in before getting into bed. Start off with a one-minute plank to give your core one last workout. Then, settle down with yoga before bed. Yoga helps clear the mind and will put you in a peaceful mood before sleeping. Try going into Tree Pose for 20 seconds, then Warrior 3 for 20 seconds, then finally end with Downward Dog for 20 seconds before lying back in Corpse Pose and nodding off to a great night's sleep.

Chapter 4 Action Summary

- Commit to doing some exercise every day.

- Do two strength-training sessions and three aerobic-focused workout each week.

- Burn more calories by building movement spurts into your entire day.

5

Add Healthy Fats to Meals

They'll satisfy your hunger so you won't overeat carbs, and the right ones are good for your heart.

IF YOU ARE OLD enough to remember when Mark Wahlberg was Marky Mark, you'll recall that it was a time when all fats were considered as terrible for your heart as boy bands were for your ears. A lot of '90s fads have come back into fashion recently, from chokers to slip dresses, but we hope fat-phobia never leaves 1992.

Eating fat doesn't make you fat. In fact, our bodies need some dietary fat to function properly. Healthy sources of fats and oils—think almonds, not chicken wings—can help you quash hunger, maximize your metabolism, lose weight, and absorb key nutrients like vitamins A, D, E, and K in broccoli (butter it up!). What's more, many of the foods with healthy fats, such as nuts, seeds, and fish, are also rich in another important nutrient—protein. By skimping on fats, you could inadvertently limit your intake of high-quality protein. Not good.

One of the reasons behind the misleading fat phobia is that each gram of fat contains nine calories, compared to just four calories per gram of carbohydrates or proteins. So, it can be easy to get more calories than you want when you eat fatty foods, even healthy fatty foods. That's why portion control becomes super important when you're planning to add healthy fats to your meals. The government's Dietary Guidelines for Americans recommends consuming about 20 to 35 percent of your daily calories from fat. That means that if you eat about 2,000 calories per day, you would eat about 400 to 700 of those calories from fat, or about 44 to 78 grams of fat.

Not all fats are created equal. While everyone knows olive oil is a healthy monounsaturated fat, some truly are downright dangerous (like the trans fats in margarines). Others are simply confusing. (Is a polyunsaturated fat good for me? And what does it look like?)

What's more, the way you use the fats really matters to your heart. For example, high-heat frying in fat creates by-products that are bad for your heart, so we're not going to recommend fried food—even if it's a vegetable fried in olive oil! Meanwhile, a little drizzle of oil on a salad is a superb choice. See, today's science suggests that an oversimplified, one-size-fits-all approach to fat is just plain wrong. To enjoy the benefits of the best fats on the 7-Day Healthy Heart Diet plan, you need to learn the basics about the fats in your food and which ones to eat more (or less) of.

Trans Fats

There is only one category of fat that should be truly avoided at all costs—industrially produced trans fats. You might see these ingredients, such as partially hydrogenated soybean oil, listed on the labels of some foods in your pantry. When certain oils, such as soybean oil or cottonseed oil, undergo a process called partial hydrogenation, they become solid at room temperature. That's a helpful attribute for food manufacturers using them as an ingredient, but studies suggest it's bad for your arteries.

When these fats float through your arteries, they contribute to the formation and rupture of dangerous fatty deposits called plaques. These plaques can clog your arteries and increase your risk of a range of heart problems, including heart attacks. A recent study published in the journal *Atherosclerosis* suggests that people with higher blood levels of trans fats have a higher risk of particularly risky types of arterial plaques.

Trans fats are so troublesome, the Food and Drug Administration mandated that all foods must be free of these fats by June 18, 2018. But some components of the deadline were extended, so it will be a few more years before industrial trans fats are completely gone from packaged foods for good. (And the action does not apply to restaurants that might be using these oils to deep-fry foods.)

Meanwhile, in May 2018, the World Health Organization (WHO) launched a global initiative called REPLACE to eliminate artificial trans fats from the world food supply by 2023. For the first time, global health officials are finally asking countries to remove the harmful oils from their foods. According to the WHO, intake of trans fats has led to more than 500,000 deaths a year from heart disease.

Further evidence of the effect of eliminating these bad fats comes from bans of trans fats in the United States. A study published in the *Journal of Health Economics* found that after eleven New York counties enacted a ban on trans fats from restaurant offerings in 2007, there was a 4.5 percent reduction in deaths related to cardiovascular disease. Another study published in *JAMA Cardiology* highlighted a significant decrease in strokes just three years after the ban was implemented.

It's important to note that while artificial trans fats will be banned from our packaged food supply, you may still see trans fats listed on nutrition labels. That's because meat and dairy products have some naturally occurring trans fats; however, research suggests that they aren't as bad for your health as industrially manufactured trans fats. Check nutrition labels to ensure there are no artificial trans fats lurking in your cupboards.

Saturated Fats

The next most infamous fat, saturated fat, is controversial. Some studies suggest that saturated fat intake is associated with a higher risk of cardiovascular disease. Others, including a recent comprehensive meta-analysis in the *Annals of Internal Medicine,* have concluded that there is no significant evidence that saturated fats increase your risks for cardiovascular diseases, and that consuming the right types of saturated fat in moderation can actually help you torch body fat. For example, it may be helpful to eat more stearic acid, a type of saturated fat found in milk, which could actually have cholesterol-lowering properties. It may be wise to eat less palmitic acid, found in palm oil and conventionally raised animal meats, which has been linked to increased cholesterol. The bottom line: If your diet is full of nutrient-rich foods consumed in reasonable portions (like the super heart foods in Chapter 3), your saturated fat consumption will likely fall within a reasonable range automatically.

Monounsaturated Fats

Monounsaturated fatty acids (MUFAs), found in olive oil, avocados, walnuts, and more, have been shown to reduce appetite and promote weight loss. They also protect your heart by helping to clear harmful LDL cholesterol from your bloodstream, according to clinical research. A recent study in the *American Journal of Clinical Nutrition* suggests that plant foods rich in MUFAs are superior to animal-based foods rich in MUFAs, such as chicken. By eating nuts, seeds, and healthy plant oils every day, you will eat more MUFAs than saturated fats, which can be helpful.

Polyunsaturated Fats

You probably know the most famous polyunsaturated fats, the omega-3 fatty acids, which come in capsule form at your local supplement store. There are actually eleven different omega-3 fatty acids, but the three must-haves for humans are ALA (alpha-linolenic acid), DHA (docosahexaenoic acid), and EPA (eicosapentaenoic acid). These fats aid in reducing inflammation, cholesterol levels, body fat, and hunger. You can find EPA and DHA in fish, such as sardines, sockeye salmon, or canned light tuna. You can find ALA in flaxseeds, chia seeds, canola oil, and more. Like all omega-3s, ALA helps to reduce appetite, control inflammation, and promote weight loss, and studies looking specifically at ALA have found it plays a role in reducing the risk of heart attacks, lowering cholesterol levels, and bringing down blood pressure.

Omega-6 fatty acids are also important, but the average American diet now has from 14 to 25 times the amount of omega-6s we really need, according to an analysis by researchers at the University of Maryland Medical Center. The researchers say that the increased consumption of linoleic acid (LA)—which is found in the vegetable oils that all our fatty foods are fried in—has been a primary driver of our increased levels of omega-6s. Too much omega-6 in your diet can lead to inflammation, overeating, weight gain, and heart disease. While omega-6s are still essential fatty acids and have a rightful place in your diet, if you're eating fried foods regularly, you'll benefit from cutting back on your intake.

The bottom line is that it's easy to eat the right fats by avoiding burgers, pizza, fried foods, and other options you won't find in our meal plan and instead fill up on nuts and seeds, eggs, dairy products, and lean meats.

The Healthy Heart Diet Goal: Consume a serving of nuts or seeds per day and two sources of good-quality dairy, eggs, meat, or fish. About a third of your daily calories should come from fats from nutritious, filling sources. We covered one of our favorite fatty foods, avocados, back in Chapter 3, since it's a fruit! Here are some other smart ways to take in the right fats.

Heart-Helper Supplements

A healthy diet will nourish your cardiovascular system, but a strategic supplement here and there may also help in certain situations. As always, it's important to check with your doctor before you pop any supplements, so ask about these:

Probiotics. These capsules of helpful bacteria are famous for their digestive benefits, but emerging evidence suggests that they might help your heart, too. In a study review, researchers from Australia found that probiotic consumption reduced systolic blood pressure by 3.56 mm Hg and diastolic blood pressure by 2.38 mm Hg. Their analysis suggests that probiotics might work best when taken for eight or more weeks, and that the product should have more than one species of bacteria and a total dose of more than 100 billion colony-forming units.

Omega-3 fatty acids (fish oil). In a 2017 science advisory, a panel of experts the American Heart Association recommended that people with coronary heart disease, such as those who have already had a heart attack, could benefit from omega-3 fatty acid supplements. Treatment is also recommended for people with prevalent heart failure without preserved left ventricular function. For people who do not already have heart disease, the jury is still out on fish oil supplements. If you are unsure if they are right for you, check with your doctor or simply get your omega-3s by eating more oily fish.

Magnesium. A study review published in the *American Journal of Clinical Nutrition* showed that people who took magnesium supplements reduced their systolic blood pressure by an average of 4.18 mm Hg and their diastolic blood pressure by an average of 2.27 mm Hg.

Garlic extract. This stinky herb has long been heralded for its cholesterol-lowering benefits, and new research from Poland suggests that garlic can do even more. People who consumed a garlic extract supplement daily for 3 months reduced not only their lipid levels but also experienced other heart-healthy benefits such as improved arterial flexibility and lower levels of C-reactive protein—a marker of inflammation.

Aspirin. First of all, this one is not technically a supplement; it's an over-the-counter drug, but a daily dose is beneficial for some people. You've probably heard that aspirin is good for your heart, and most doctors agree that it's a must-have for people who have already suffered a heart attack. For people looking to prevent a heart attack, aspirin may or may not be worth it, the experts say. Aspirin's blood-thinning, anti-inflammatory, heart-boosting benefits have to be weighed against its risks, namely the risk of gastrointestinal bleeding. Ask your doctor to help you weigh the options.

SNACK ON NUTS AND SEEDS

Squirrel away some nuts. People who eat one serving of nuts 5 or more days a week have a 14 percent reduced risk of cardiovascular disease, suggests research published in the *Journal of the American College of Cardiology*. The healthy fats, fiber, minerals, and antioxidants in nuts may help you control your blood sugar, reduce your cholesterol, and more. Seeds like flaxseeds and chia seeds contain many similarly beneficial nutrients. Aim for a serving of nuts and/or seeds per day, which is about a handful of nuts or seeds or 2 tablespoons of nut or seed butter. That's right, nut butter counts, as long as it is isn't packed with a bunch of sugar, salt, fillers, and added oils. Consider these options.

Almonds

Simply popping a few almonds in your mouth could help you shed pounds, and not just because almonds are better for you than, say, candy. A study published in the *Journal of the American Heart Association* found that eating 1.5 ounces of almonds a day helped people reduce belly and leg fat. And another study of overweight adults found that people who ate ¼ cup of almonds for 6 months had a 62 percent greater reduction in weight and BMI. Almonds have lots of good fats and also boast more protein than some other nuts, making them a filling choice for snacks.

Try Justin's Maple Almond Butter or Manna Organics Manna Butter–Sprouted Almond Espresso with fruit slices or vegetable sticks.

Chia Seeds

Tiny chia seeds—yes, the same ones in your Chia Pet from the '90s—pack a nutritional wallop. They're loaded with essential nutrients like omega-3s, calcium, potassium, and magnesium. Chia also packs an impressive 3 grams of protein and 5 grams of hunger-crushing fiber per tablespoon. And since the seeds form a gel when mixed with water (they can hold up to ten times their weight in liquid), they digest slowly, making them a powerful force against the munchies—which is great news for those looking to control portions and cravings. Sprinkle 'em on sweet potatoes or on fruit with nut butter.

Flaxseeds

A mere tablespoon of these ultra-powerful seeds serves up nearly 3 grams of belly-filling fiber for just 55 calories. We like that ratio. Not to mention, flaxseeds are the richest plant source of omega-3 fats, which help reduce inflammation, ward off mood swings, and help prevent heart disease and diabetes. A diet of heart-healthy fats like those found in flaxseeds raises good (HDL) cholesterol levels. Flaxseeds make a subtle, nutty addition to smoothies, salad dressings, and yogurt. But you'll need *ground* flaxseeds in order to get all the heart benefits; the solid seeds aren't easily digested.

Try NuttZo Organic 7 Nut & Seed Butter for a mix of nuts and seeds.

Pistachios

This is a nut you want to start eating by the handful, *literally*. Pistachios contain fewer calories but more potassium and vitamin K than any other nut in the market. A one-ounce serving of dry-roasted pistachios contains just 160 calories, yet packs six grams of protein, three grams of fiber, and 15 grams of fat. For comparison, cashews only contain 16 to 18 nuts per one-ounce serving, whereas pistachios are able to squeeze a whopping 49 nuts (with the shell removed, that is) into that miniscule 1-ounce measure.

Walnuts

Perhaps this is Mother Nature's way of giving us a hint: These nuts, which have a heart shape, are brimming in antioxidants and omega-3 fatty acids that can significantly reduce the risk of heart disease—an umbrella term that refers to a number of deadly complications (including heart attack and stroke) that account for about 600,000 deaths in the United States annually. The most comprehensive review of clinical trials on nut consumption in relation to cardiovascular disease showed consuming just 1 ounce of walnuts five or more times a week—about a handful every day—can slash heart disease risk by nearly 40 percent! Most of the nuts' heart-health benefits come from walnut oil, so release the oils by roasting them in a dry pan over medium heat. Or pick up a bottle of walnut oil for dressing and cooking.

DON'T DISCOUNT DAIRY

And don't limit yourself to the skim variety. People who eat a lot of high-fat dairy actually have the lowest incidence of diabetes, according to a 2015 study of 26,930 people published in the *American Journal of Clinical Nutrition.* (And diabetes and heart disease are often linked.) By contrast, people in the study who ate a lot of low-fat dairy products had the highest incidence. The researchers speculated that while the calcium, protein, vitamin D, and other nutrients in yogurt (the dairy product studied) are good for us, we need the fat that goes along with them in order to get their protective effects. Try these:

Protein-packed Cheeses

Per calorie, low-fat mozzarella and cottage cheese are two of the best high-protein foods, and they're versatile enough to pair with other foods. After an iron-pumping workout, you want to eat a snack that's full of energy-restoring carbs as well as muscle-building protein, so try cottage cheese on top of rye bread and avocado or mozzarella with a slice of tomato and basil. We love Good Culture Cottage Cheese. Each classic container has 150 calories, 6 g fat (3.5 g saturated fat), 450 mg sodium, 4 g carbs, and 19 g protein.

Yogurt

A study of more than 2,000 adults revealed that those who consume just 2 percent of their total daily calories from yogurt—that would be like eating one 6-ounce cup of yogurt every 3 days—have a 31 percent lower incidence of hypertension than those who eat the creamy stuff less often, according to the American Heart Association. And another study found that each weekly serving of yogurt was associated with a 6 percent reduction in one's risk of hypertension. It goes back to those two essential nutrients, vitamin D and calcium. Some yogurts also provide potassium, a proven blood-pressure reducer. An 8-ounce container of Stonyfield's Organic Smooth & Creamy yogurt, for example, contains up to 11 percent of the day's recommended intake of D and calcium, more than you'd get from a small banana. Just keep an eye out for flavored yogurts—they are usually packed with added sugars. (More on that on page 111.)

EAT THE RIGHT MEATS AND EGGS

In this book, we recommend a primarily plant-based diet, but that doesn't mean you have to go full-on vegan or vegetarian. Eggs are a welcome source of protein, as are many meats. Just start thinking of meat as a side dish instead of the main event in a meal, and choose fresh cuts of meat, not highly processed ones. When you want beef, choose grass-fed varieties. They contain higher levels of omega-3 fatty acids, nutrients that have been shown to reduce the risk of heart disease, than conventionally grown meats, according to a study published in *Nutrition Journal*. At the same time, consider fish to be a critical part of a heart-healthy diet: The American Heart Association recommends eating fish, especially fatty fish, at least two times per week. Choose from among these heart-healthy favorites:

Eggs

Let's clear something up right off the bat: You do not need to avoid eggs to have a heart-healthy diet. Once maligned for their cholesterol content, eggs are now accepted as one of the best delivery vehicles for filling protein, and it turns out that the cholesterol in eggs is not a problem. (Cholesterol in food doesn't necessarily translate to cholesterol in the arteries, scientists now say.) Eggs are also the top dietary source of choline, which attacks the gene mechanism that triggers your body to store fat around your liver.

When shopping for eggs, you might have noticed that there are more labels on egg cartons than you used to see. Although "free range," "pasture raised," "antibiotic free," and "cage free" are labels you'll commonly see on eggs, their meanings are misleading. *Cage free* does mean the chickens aren't living in cages, but it doesn't necessarily mean they're any better off. Oftentimes, these chickens live solely indoors and have little room to move freely. Instead, look for "Certified Humane Free Range." According to the Humane Farm Animal Care (HFAC), a nonprofit certification organization dedicated to improving the lives of farm animals, this certification means that each chicken has two square feet of space and hens must be outdoors for at least six hours daily, if the weather permits. Another one to watch for is "Certified Humane Pasture Raised," which means that the hens that produce the eggs have at least 108 square feet to roam around and are outdoors year-round in fields that are rotated. The hens can also go inside in the evening to take shelter from predators or inclement weather.

Halibut

You already knew that fish is rich in protein, but you might be surprised to learn that halibut beats fiber-rich oatmeal and vegetables in the satiety department. The Satiety Index of Common Foods, an Australian study published in the *European Journal of Clinical Nutrition,* ranks it as the number two most filling food—bested only by boiled potatoes for its ability to fill you satisfactorily. A separate Australian study that compared the satiety of different animal proteins found a nutritionally similar white fish (flake) to be significantly more satiating than beef and chicken; feelings of satiety after a meal of the white fish also declined at a much slower rate. Study authors attribute the filling factor of white fish like halibut to its impressive protein content and influence on serotonin, one of the key hormones responsible for appetite signals.

Pork

Once considered an enemy of doctors and dieters, pork has been coming around as a healthier alternative of late—as long as you choose the right cut. Your best bet is pork tenderloin: A University of Wisconsin Study found that a 3-ounce serving of pork tenderloin has 24 grams of protein and 83 milligrams of waist-whittling choline (in the latter case, about the same as a medium egg). In a study published in the journal *Nutrients,* scientists asked 144 overweight people to eat a diet rich in fresh lean pork. After 3 months, the pork-eating group saw a significant reduction in waist size, BMI, and belly fat, with no accompanying reduction in muscle mass. The researchers speculate that the amino acid profile of pork protein may contribute to greater fat burning.

Poultry

Turkey is rich in the omega-3 DHA (docosahexaenoic acid)

—18 milligrams per serving—which has been shown to boost brain function, improve your mood, and turn off fat genes, preventing fat cells from growing in size. Just make sure you buy white meat only; dark contains too much fat and too many calories to have the effect. And know that you're doing your health a double solid by grilling at home: Restaurant versions can be packed with fatty add-ins to increase flavor. Meanwhile, chicken packs a whopping 26 grams of protein per 3-ounce breast.

Salmon

Add a fillet of this fish to your diet just twice a week to get the amount of heart-healthy omega-3 fatty acids recommended by the American Heart Association. Healthy people aren't the only ones who can reap the rewards of salmon as a dinner choice; even people who are already at a high risk of cardiovascular disease can get a leg up by serving up some salmon a couple of times a week. Omega-3s reduce the risk of arrhythmia, they decrease triglyceride levels, and they can actually slightly lower blood pressure. Just make sure you pick wild salmon, which has been proved to be significantly lower in cancer-linked PCBs.

Tuna

As a prime source of protein and DHA, canned light tuna is one of the best and most affordable fish for weight loss. While you'll find two types of fatty acids in cold-water fish and fish oils—DHA and eicosapentaenoic acid (EPA)— researchers say DHA can be 40 to 70 percent more effective than EPA at down-regulating fat genes in the abdomen, preventing belly fat cells from expanding in size. But what about the toxic mercury that can be found in fatty fish?

Mercury levels in tuna vary by species; generally speaking, the larger and leaner the fish, the higher the mercury level. Bluefin and albacore rank among the most toxic varieties, according to a study in *Biology Letters*. But canned chunk light tuna, harvested from the smallest fish, is considered a "low-mercury fish" and can be enjoyed two to three times a week (up to 12 ounces), according to the FDA's most recent guidelines.

COOK WITH HEALTHIER OILS

Whether you're searing a steak or dressing a salad, a splash of oil can make a dish. We say that cooking with oil is a beautiful thing, as long as you choose the right kinds and you don't deep-fry with them. Oils give dishes flavor, which can help you feel satisfied with smaller portions of foods. Plus, a little bit of fat on a salad or vegetables can actually help your body absorb certain nutrients, such as vitamins A, C, and E, more effectively. Try the following kinds; just drizzle carefully, since a serving size is 1 teaspoon.

Avocado Oil

Made from pressed avocados, this oil is rich in heart-healthy monounsaturated fats that may help improve cholesterol and ward off hunger. It also contains vitamins B and E and potassium. The oil has a mild nutty taste and a light avocado aroma. It works well drizzled over breads, fish, and homemade pizzas. It also pairs nicely with watermelon, grapefruit, and oranges. Add some to your fruit salad to create a new twist on a classic dish.

Canola Oil

Canola, derived from the seeds of a plant in the broccoli family, comes in toward the top of our list with its near-perfect 2.5:1 ratio of omega-6 to omega-3 fats. It's also rich in alpha-linolenic acid (ALA), an essential omega-3 fatty acid that a recent study suggests may play a role in weight maintenance. This is the best option for everyday cooking situations. Canola oil can withstand relatively high levels of heat, and its flavor is fairly neutral, so it won't dominate a dish.

Extra-Virgin Olive Oil

Extra-virgin olive oil may increase blood levels of serotonin, a hormone associated with satiety. Plus, olive oil is also loaded with polyphenols, antioxidants that help battle many diseases such as cancer and osteoporosis and conditions that lead to brain deterioration. Expensive extra-virgin, with its robust flavor, should be saved to dress salads, vegetables, and cooked dishes. For cooking purposes, regular or light olive oil is sufficient.

Flaxseed Oil

Also known as linseed oil—yes, the stuff you used in art class—this fat contains ALA, an essential omega-3 fatty acid that can aid weight maintenance and may reduce heart disease risks by promoting blood vessel health and reducing inflammation. Flaxseed oil doesn't hold up well when exposed to heat so don't plan to sauté with it. Drizzle it on top of salads or use it instead of olive oil or mayo when whipping up pestos, tuna salads, and sauces. Or pour it into a smoothie!

Macadamia Nut Oil

You might have to hunt around in the specialty stores for it, but this bold and buttery oil may be the healthiest you'll find: Eighty-four percent of the fat in macadamia nuts is monounsaturated, and it has a very high percentage of omega-3 fatty acids. It's also a source of phytosterols, plant-derived compounds that have been associated with decreased cholesterol levels. Due to its medium to high smoke point, macadamia nut oil is best suited for baking, stir-frying, and oven cooking. For a quick snack, toss slices of sweet potatoes with the nut oil and bake them in the oven at 350°F for 20 minutes, or until crispy.

Peanut Oil

Peanut oil is loaded with a monounsaturated fat called oleic acid (OEA) that can help reduce appetite and promote weight loss. Because of its high smoke point, peanut oil should be your go-to oil for high-heat tasks like wok-cooking and pan-searing.

Walnut Oil

Recently making a splash on restaurant menus and grocery store shelves, this oil has a rich, nutty roasted flavor. A small Penn State study found that a diet rich in walnuts and walnut oil may help the body respond better to stress, and can also help keep diastolic blood pressure levels down. Walnut oil is also rich in polyunsaturated fatty acids that may increase diet-induced calorie burn and resting metabolic rate (the rate at which we use calories to keep our heart pumping and our body running). And walnuts have more omega-3 fatty acids than any other nut. Mix with sherry vinegar, olive oil, cumin, and a pinch of salt and pepper to make a salad dressing. This oil doesn't do well under heat, so it shouldn't be used for hot-surface cooking or high-temperature baking.

Chapter 5 Action Summary

- Don't fear fats. Do understand the different types and the benefits of each.

- Use fats in meals for flavor and to keep you feeling full longer, to help clobber cravings.

- Try (very hard) to eat at least two servings of fish every week.

- Snack on seeds and nuts. Focus on walnuts, one of the healthiest you can eat.

6

Avoid High-Sodium Foods

Reducing salt in your diet could do your heart some big favors.

READY FOR A FISH STORY? It's about our friend Jim, who's fifty-one and on the heavy side. There's heart disease in his family. His dad, a longtime smoker, died of congestive heart failure a few years back. At seventy-three, his mother has high blood pressure and diabetes and uses a walker. Jim's blood pressure is bordering on high, too, but he's not yet on medicine. He wants to bring his BP down with diet and exercise, and he's gotten pretty disciplined about both. Kudos, Jim! He also started taking fish oil capsules daily and eating fish twice a week, as he is tonight at the Japanese restaurant in town.

Jim ordered tuna, salmon, and mackerel sushi—all good sources of heart-healthy omega-3 fatty acids. He even requested the healthier brown rice instead of white and ordered an unsweetened iced tea to wash it down. But here's where well-intentioned Jim went wrong: He used his chopsticks to dunk every bite of sushi in a bath of soy sauce. A single tablespoon of soy sauce contains 1,000 milligrams (mg) of sodium, and Jim filled his shallow soy sauce bowl several times, meaning he consumed more than his recommended daily limit of 1,500 mg in one meal.

When it comes to sodium, condiments are bad news. A serious squirt of ketchup contains 160 mg. Mustard, 55. A tablespoon of teriyaki sauce, 610. If you are trying to watch your sodium intake, putting down the salt shaker isn't enough. You have to recognize which foods and flavor enhancers (like soy sauce) are brimming with sodium so you can avoid them. It takes effort, but salt reduction is critical for good heart health.

WHAT HAPPENS WHEN YOU EAT SALT

Our bodies need sodium to function properly. About 500 mg per day is required to maintain a healthy fluid balance and keep your muscles and nerves working well. However, your kidneys take a hit when you eat sodium in excess. One of the kidneys' jobs is to process the sodium you eat. But when your kidneys can't clear all the salt, say, after you down a plate of buffalo wings and french fries, some of the sodium ends up in your bloodstream. There, it causes your body to hold on to more fluid, raising the volume of blood in your vessels and applying greater pressure against their walls.

"There is generally a direct relationship between higher dietary sodium consumption and raised blood pressure," says Andrew Moran, MD, MPH, assistant professor of medicine at Columbia University Medical Center.

So, if you need sodium to survive but not enough to cause damage, how do you strike a healthy balance? It takes some detective work. First, figure out how much salt you already eat on an average day. Since three-quarters of our sodium intake comes from processed foods, that's a good place to start your sleuthing. Think about what you ate yesterday, look up the nutrition facts, and add up the sodium. You might be surprised. If you have a history of heart disease or have been diagnosed with high blood pressure, then your doctor may encourage you to follow the American Heart Association's guidelines: no more than 2,300 mg—that's about 1 teaspoon—per day, with an ideal limit of 1,500 mg per day. The average American eats more about 3,400 mg of sodium per day, much more than the AHA recommends.

"Curbing sodium intake does lower blood pressure, and for people with hypertension, it can help their blood pressure-lowering medications to work better," says Dr. Moran.

Walk away from hypertension

Regular physical activity—adding up to, say, 150 minutes a week, which is about 30 minutes most days of the week—can lower your blood pressure by 5 to 8 mm Hg.

To stay within the AHA's guidelines, you'll need to read the sodium numbers on nutrition labels very carefully. A food journal app or online food tracker can help you add up your daily milligrams of salt.

When you don't prepare your food yourself, assume that you're taking in a fair amount of salt. The average restaurant entrée contains 1,286 mg of sodium, more than half the AHA's recommended daily limit, suggests new research published in the *American Journal of Preventive Medicine*. Of all meal categories, salads had the least salt.

Now, if you don't have blood pressure problems, then you might not need to be quite as strict about your sodium intake. However, it's still smart to pay attention. One British study found that for every additional 1,000 milligrams of sodium (a little less than ½ teaspoon) you eat a day, your risk of obesity spikes by 25 percent. One problem is that salty food can be so satisfying that it's hard to stop eating it, contributing to excessive calorie intake. Obesity is hard on your heart.

A caveat: If you are a competitive athlete, you work out hard and sweat a lot, or you have a job that exposes you to major heat stress and sweating, then you probably lose a lot of salt through sweat on an average day. You might need to eat a little more salt than the rest of us, so consult a dietitian or your doctor for tailored advice.

Your Healthy Heart Diet Goal: Assess your salt intake and bring it into the healthy zone—2,300 mg of sodium per day or, ideally, 1,500 mg or less for those with risk factors. By eating more whole, minimally processed foods, you can effortlessly reduce your sodium intake. In the meantime, watch your intake of the following salt-packed foods.

Bagels

Depending on which type you pick up, you can get a whopping 600 mg of sodium in just one fluffy carb pillow—and that's *before* adding a smear of cream cheese. Eek! When struck with a bagel craving, opt for a bagel thin or a Bantam bagel. These doughnut hole–size bagels are filled with cream cheese and still manage to be lower in calories and sodium than a normal-size bagel.

Canned Vegetables

Veggies may be a cornerstone of a blood pressure–friendly diet, but canned ones aren't the best choice. The preservatives and sauces that keep the vitamin-filled vegetables company inside the container are packed with sodium. Look for "no salt added" or "low sodium" options, and be sure to rinse your veggies thoroughly before digging in. Can't find an unsalted option? Consider switching to frozen vegetables; there are plenty of unsalted selections. And if you use canned beans, rinse them before using in a recipe.

Capers

When it comes to your blood pressure and heart health, condiments matter. Those capers atop your Chicken Piccata? They carry more than 200 mg of salt per *tablespoon*.

Cheese-smothered Appetizers

In Chapter 5, we mentioned that a little cheese here and there is OK. But that doesn't mean you should order all the fried, cheese-drenched nachos and other sodium-packed (and calorie-laden) restaurant offerings you can imagine. Case in point: Arby's Mozzarella Sticks contain 1,570 mg of sodium in just four pieces.

Fried Foods

You should be wary of fried foods because of their excessive content of potentially dangerous fats. But it just so happens that many fried foods are also swollen with sodium. Take the House Sampler from Buffalo Wild Wings as an example: With nachos, beer-battered onion rings, mozzarella sticks, and boneless wings and sauces to dress them, this is a bona fide sodium smorgasbord weighing in at 5,550 mg of sodium. It also has 2,480 calories. Then there's Applebee's Double Crunch Shrimp. This meal packs 3,700 mg of sodium, in addition to too many calories (1,320) for one meal.

Frozen Dinners

Sure, they're quick and easy to prepare, but frozen dinners can have some drawbacks, including more sodium than you'd expect. Even the healthy-sounding options can be surprisingly salty. Two prime examples: Lean Cuisine's Baked Chicken contains 720 mg of sodium but only 260 calories. To fill up, you'd probably need to eat more food with the meal that could possibly even push the sodium content even higher. Special K's Sausage, Egg & Cheese Flatbread Breakfast Sandwich carries 700 mg—or just under half a day's worth of sodium. When you're in the freezer aisle, look for meals with less than 500 mg of sodium per serving.

Jerky

Jerky is trendy right now, thanks in part to the ever-growing Paleo trend. Sure, it's free of refined grains and packed with protein, but it's also notoriously high in salt—not good news if you have high blood pressure or want to keep your heart healthy. A small (1-ounce) serving can have upward of 700 mg of salt, which is more than four times what you'd find in a 1-ounce serving of chips. If you're snacking on jerky after a hard, sweaty workout, that's one thing. If you're sitting in front of the TV with a bagful, you might need to reconsider your life choices.

Pasta Sauce

Want some pasta with that salt!? A half cup of Hunt's Tomato Sauce packs 820 mg of sodium—which is more than you'd find in 96 Cheez-It crackers. Look for jars of tomato sauce with fewer than 350 mg per ½-cup serving. Both Amy's Light in Sodium Organic Family Marinara and Ragu Light No Sugar Added Tomato & Basil fit the bill. And when restaurants add the sauces, watch out. Olive Garden's Tour of Italy boasts an estimated 3,250 mg of sodium per meal.

Pizza

Almost every ingredient in pizza has the potential to be salty, from the crust to the sauce to the cheese to the toppings. If you buy a premade pizza packed with pepperoni, you could hit your salt quota in just one meal. For example, Red Baron Thin & Crispy Pepperoni Pizza contains 1,010 mg sodium per serving, which, by the way, is just one-third of the pizza. If you make it from scratch using homemade low-salt dough, fresh mozzarella, and fresh tomatoes, you can enjoy pizza without the salt guilt.

Processed Meats

For centuries, humans have been curing meats to preserve them. But in the twenty-first century, we have refrigeration, and we eat ham and bacon just because they are delicious. Yes, your taste buds may rejoice when you eat processed meats, but your heart—well, let's just say if it had a personality it would cringe. In a study published in *Public Health Nutrition*, every daily serving of processed meat increased people's risk of death from heart disease by 15 percent. The high salt content in processed meats can be problematic, and many processed meats also contain nitrites, preservatives that can break down into more harmful substances called N-nitroso compounds. We wouldn't dare suggest that you can never ever eat bacon again, but can you save it for special occasions?

Restaurant Soup

Get this: P.F. Chang's Hot & Sour Soup Bowl packs an artery-shivering 9,590 mg of sodium. That's more than 4 days' worth, or the equivalent of about 55—yes, 55—individual bags of Cool Ranch Doritos. Not all restaurants' bowls of broth are quite *that* salt-filled, but even chains like Ruby Tuesday and Applebee's don't ladle out anything with less than half a day's sodium per bowl. Canned soups are often sodium-packed, too, so check the label before indulging. For example, Progresso New England Clam Chowder packs 1,780 mg in every 2 cups. Soups can be a great addition to a heart-healthy diet when you make them from scratch with low-sodium broth. Check out our recipes in Chapter 10.

Sandwiches

According to a *Journal of the Academy of Nutrition and Dietetics* study, nearly half of Americans consume a sandwich every day. The bread and condiments certainly don't help the salt situation, but cold cuts and cheese are the primary culprits, contributing about 250 mg of sodium per slice. And let's be real: We all use at least three or four slices of the stuff in our sandwiches, which equates to 1,000 mg of salt in a single sitting. And when you leave it to restaurants to portion out these meats, you can really end up in a pickle. For example, the Quiznos Classic Italian 12-inch Sandwich contains 4,150 mg of sodium! When you craft sandwiches at home, start with Ezekiel 4:9 Low Sodium Sprouted Whole Grain Bread. Pile on veggies or smear the bread with avocado for extra flavor sans salt.

Soy Sauce

We love a good, veggie-packed stir fry, but make sure you pick low-sodium soy sauce instead of the regular variety. A mere tablespoon of regular soy sauce has almost half a day's worth of sodium, but some low-sodium types have half that.

The Power of Potassium

To counteract excess sodium, call upon its adversary—potassium. This mineral works against sodium in several important ways and can help you regulate your blood pressure. It's recommended that adults get 4,700 milligrams of potassium per day, but the average person eats just a bit more than half of that. Bananas are famously packed with potassium, 422 mg worth, but you can also find this mineral in the following foods:

Cooked Mushrooms

555 mg of potassium per 1 cup sliced

No need to splurge on exotic 'shrooms; new research proves the humble white button mushroom has as much potassium—in some cases, more—and antioxidant properties as expensive varieties.

Cooked Spinach

839 mg of potassium per 1 cup

It's hard to eat too much spinach. Stock up on a few bags at the beginning of the week and challenge yourself to sneak it into every meal. A handful of raw greens in one of your healthy smoothies? You'll never taste it!

White Beans

595 mg of potassium per ½ cup cooked

Dried beans tend to be slightly higher in fiber and slightly lower on the glycemic index than canned. For convenience, though, canned varieties are usually fine and can help break down some of the beans' gas-causing oligosaccharides; just check the label for additives like sugar, and rinse away the liquid the beans are packed in thoroughly before enjoying.

Winter Squash

896 mg of potassium per 1 cup baked

There are numerous varieties of squash, and all provide a healthy dose of potassium. Squash tastes best in its peak season, so let the "fresh test" be your guide, and choose whatever looks, smells, and feels prime for picking at the market.

Natural solutions

Recent studies have found simple, natural ways to lower blood pressure. Give them a try.

Grow good bacteria. A serving of probiotic-rich foods like yogurt, sauerkraut, or kefir daily for 8 weeks has been shown to lower systolic blood pressure by 3.5 points.

Get outside. Thirty-minutes of exposure to the sun's UV rays can dilate blood vessels, temporarily lowering BP.

Sip a cuppa tea. In an experiment, people who were asked to sip three 8-ounce cups of hibiscus tea every day lowered their systolic blood pressure by an average of 7 points over six weeks.

Chapter 6 Action Summary

- Identify hidden sources of sodium in your diet. (Read nutrition labels.)
- Don't eat out at restaurants as much.
- Eat more potassium-rich foods.
- You are following Chapter 4's exercise plan, right?

Trim Added Sugars from Your Diet

Replace fast-burning carbs with foods that'll supply you with lasting energy.

CARBS SOMETIMES get a bad reputation, but they don't all deserve it. They're important energy sources for your body, and many foods rich in carbohydrates, like fruits and vegetables, are perfectly healthy. The foods to be wary of are the ones loaded with fiber-free, processed carbs, such as sugar and white flour.

Your body metabolizes these fiber-free starches and sugars quickly, leaving you hungry in short order and contributing to weight gain, insulin resistance, and other heart-damaging problems, over time. In contrast, when you eat carbs that have a good amount of fiber, which your body can't convert to sugar, you may feel fuller longer and end up eating less.

Make added sugars the first simple carbs on your hit list. Research published in *BMJ Open* suggests that Americans eat an average of 18 teaspoons of added sugars per day. That's double the maximum recommended for men by the American Heart Association. What's more, almost 90 percent of that sweetness comes from "ultra-processed foods" like soft drinks, fruit drinks, breads, cakes, cookies, pies, desserts, sweet snacks, ice cream and ice pops, breakfast cereals, and milk-based drinks with added sugar. It may be obvious that these aren't exactly healthy choices but even if you avoid soda and decline the office doughnuts, added sugars can still sneak into your diet. It's likely they are lurking in your fridge, pantry, and freezer—and really, just about everywhere food is served. Many processed foods that seem healthy, such as peanut butter, some protein bars, and whole-wheat bread, contain added sugar in the form of syrups, nectars, honey, and other ingredients ending in "-ose."

To find (and avoid) added sugars in these manufactured foods, read the ingredients list carefully, and don't just scan the label for the word "sugar." Sugar has many alter egos. Look for ingredients like glucose, fructose, high-fructose corn syrup, dextrose, maltose, invert sugar, and more. Remember that ingredients are listed in order of quantity— so if a sugar ingredient is one of the first few listed, you might want to look for another product. The "sugars" info on the nutrition label is also helpful, although the number generally includes both natural and added sugars. If your food contains a lot of sugars on the ingredients list, there's a good chance that much of the sugar count comes from added sugars. Some food labels also list "added sugars" underneath the total sugar count. Know that four grams of added sugars equals a teaspoon.

Your Healthy Heart Diet Goal: Keep the amount of added sugars you eat in a day to less than 6teaspoons of added sugar per day (for women) or 9 teaspoons a day (for men.) At the same time, eat fewer refined grains and more whole grains—at least three servings per day. The right carbs can make up 45 to 65 percent of your daily calories. Take a look at the following foods.

Canned Fruit

Fresh fruit has natural sugars from fructose, but canned fruit often comes with extra sugar because it's packed in sugary syrup. A 1-cup serving of canned peaches, for example, can contain upward of 39 grams of sugar. If you're steering clear of fresh fruit because you need your fruit to last longer, head to the freezer aisle and reach for no-sugar-added varieties that were flash-frozen at the peak of their ripeness.

Coffee

A cup of coffee is fine by itself. But do you really begin your morning with a cup of joe, or is it more like a cup of cream and sugar? Many popular coffee drinks are absolute sugar bombs. Take the White Chocolate Mocha from Starbucks. A grande with 2 percent milk and whipped cream has twice as much sugar as a woman should eat in an entire day. Black coffee is the smartest pick, but if you can't stomach it, add the minimum amount of cream and sugar you can tolerate.

For example, at Starbucks, opt for the Nitro Cold Brew with Sweet Cream, which contains less than 1 teaspoon of sugar. Now, if you pick up bottled coffee drinks at the grocery store, exercise caution. These glass-encased beverages may be missing whipped cream and caramel drizzle, but they're far from innocent. Gold Peak's Salted Caramel Cold Brew, for example, has 53 grams of sugar. I personally like La Colombe's Draft Latte—plain, not a flavored variety—since it contains no added sugars.

Cold Cereal

Resist the nostalgia and let sugary cereals be just a childhood memory. Spooning out a bowl of Honey Smacks before school might have been fun in elementary school, but it wasn't doing you any favors then and it won't do you any now. Although the box describes it as "sweetened puffed wheat cereal," Honey Smacks should be called something like "sweetener with some puffed wheat." Sugar is the top ingredient on its list.

The best cereals are low in sugar and high in whole grains, which we'll talk more about in a bit. We recommend looking for a cereal with at least 3 grams (g) of fiber and no more than 10 g of sugar per 1-cup serving. Try Erewhon Harvest Medley, which has 0 g sugar per cup, or Barbara's Puffins Cereal, which has 5 g per ¾ cup.

Condiments and Sauces

Your favorite flavor enhancer might be more like a candy glaze. The first ingredient in Kraft Barbecue Sauce's list, for example, is sugar! A 2-tablespoon serving packs 13 grams of sugar, and I know I would have a hard time keeping it to just one serving. Read labels on sauces and keep in mind that mustard is usually a safe bet—unless it's honey mustard, of course. Also, portion size can be difficult to track when you dole things out by the squeeze. Squeeze slowly. Keep this in mind at restaurants, too. And watch for sauces that are precooked with a dish. For example, P.F. Chang's Stir-Fried Eggplant might sound healthy, but it's coated in a sauce with 41 grams of sugar. Stick to the Buddha's Feast instead.

Desserts

We probably don't need to explain why cookies, cakes, ice cream, and other indulgent treats should be reserved for special occasions, but just in case you need a reminder: These foods are typically packed with sugar. If you visit the dessert bar at a wedding, fine. But if your kitchen is well stocked with cakes, cookies, pies, and ice cream all the time, well, that's a problem. If you keep these foods in your house, you will eat them. Guaranteed.

Get rid of them to avoid temptation or pick up a few less-sugary indulgences instead to satisfy your sweet tooth with minimal added sugars. We like FlapJacked Mighty Muffin S'Mores. They contain 20 grams of muscle-building protein and an impressive 5 grams of filling fiber, thanks to oat flour and protein powder, but just 10 grams of sugar per one giant muffin. (A typical large blueberry muffin from a

FOOD FACT

2

Regular physical activity—adding up to, say, 150 minutes a week, which is about 30 minutes most days of the week—can lower your blood pressure by 5 to 8 mm Hg.

bakery has 44 grams of sugar.) Or try a Kashi Chocolate Almond Butter Cookie. The bulk of these cookies is made up of nutritious whole grains like triticale (a wheat-rye hybrid) and buckwheat, a slow-burning grain-like fruit seed. Each cookie has just 7 grams of sugar, whereas a typical chocolate cookie might have nearly double that.

Energy Drinks

These might seem harmless enough, especially if you need to push your way through a long car ride or a hard workout. But one can of Red Bull contains 27 grams of sugar—more than you'd find in six Dunkin' sugar-raised doughnuts. Coffee and tea can offer a calorie-free (or lightly sweetened) caffeine kick, plus they are naturally packed with anti-inflammatory compounds that may help your heart.

Flavored Water

Look closely at the label because flavored waters are pretty much flavored with sugar. Take Vitaminwater, for example. How much are you willing to sacrifice for a hearty helping of vitamins B and C? Glugging back just one Kiwi Strawberry Vitaminwater will get you your entire daily dose, but it comes at the expense of 32 waist-widening grams of sugar. And don't think that's all coming from natural sources like juiced fruits—the second ingredient listed on the label is crystalline fructose, and the next is cane sugar. Don't let this much added sugar sneak by you just because these drinks are marketed as healthy products.

Frozen Meals

Many packaged frozen meals come with a surprisingly high payload of sugar. Take the Healthy Choice Cafe Steamers

Sweet and Sour Chicken. Although the meal contains only 390 calories, it has 18 grams of added sugars. That's 4.5 teaspoons, or 75 percent of the daily maximum amount of added sugars for women recommended by the American Heart Association.

Fruit Drinks

Even the best drinkable fruit—100 percent juice—is inferior to fruit in whole form. But if you really want to sip your fruit, stick with 100 percent juice, not a cocktail of juice and sugar. Fruit drinks can be more sugar than juice. Take Welch's Fruit Punch Juice Drink: The number one ingredient is water, followed by high-fructose corn syrup, and *then* fruit juices. That means a good portion of this drink's 29 grams of sugar comes from added sugars, not naturally occurring fruit sugars.

Milk Alternatives

Although cow's milk contains natural sugar from lactose, the sugar in nondairy milk is often the added kind. And at 19 grams per cup, chocolate soy milk really pushes the sugar boundary. Many almond milks have added sugars, too. The bottom line: Don't assume that every alterna-milk is healthy. If you're looking for dairy alternatives, opt for unsweetened or lightly sweetened varieties.

Protein Bars

Some popular bars have more sugar than a candy bar! Take the Power Bar Performance Energy Bar in Cookie Dough, for example. The number one ingredient in this little bar is cane invert syrup, another moniker for sugar! Instead, try a Mint Chocolate RXBar, which has no added sugars.

Soda

Pop is the top source of added sugar in the average American's diet, and its colossal sugar payload goes down especially easy. Example: One 12-ounce can of Pepsi is packed with 41 grams of added sugars. You'd have to suck on 12 Werther's Originals candies to take in that much sweetness by other means!

All that sugar is hard on your heart. Having one 12-ounce soda a day raises your risk of a heart attack by 20 percent, according to a study published in the American Heart Association journal *Circulation*. The researchers found the correlation to be independent of weight factors like obesity and weight gain alone, and they believe soda's inflammatory properties play a role. Sugary beverages have also been linked to higher levels of triglycerides and low levels of HDL, or good cholesterol, which all lead to poor heart function.

Unfortunately, diet soda is no angel, either. Regular consumption of the artificial sweeteners in these carbonated "zero sugar" drinks is associated with weight gain and cardiometabolic risk, according to a meta-analysis in the *Canadian Medical Association Journal*. The best thing to drink when you're thirsty is simple H_2O. According to researchers from Loma Linda University, drinking at least five cups of water a day can cut your heart disease risk by up to 60 percent.

Soup

You know that canned soup is packed with salt (as we discussed in Chapter 6), but you may not know that many varieties are riddled with sugar, too. Campbell's Slow Kettle Style Tomato & Sweet Basil Bisque, for example, has 24 grams of sugar per cup. Sure, some of that is coming from the tomatoes, but sugar is the fourth ingredient, which just seems unnecessary.

Yogurt

It's a heart-healthy food, as we mentioned on page 81. However, some yogurts are packed with enough sugar that they should really be considered desserts. Same goes for restaurant yogurt parfaits like the Au Bon Pain Blueberry Yogurt and Wild Blueberry Parfait. It packs 48 grams of sugar, thanks to a combo of corn syrup, brown sugar, and maple syrup.

To minimize added sugar in yogurt, pick up the plain variety and add your own fruit and nuts. If you're buying something premixed, try Siggi's 4 percent Whole-Milk Skyr, Mixed Berries. Siggi's flavors this yogurt with real berries and just a hint of cane sugar, making it just 8 grams of sugar per serving.

UPGRADE YOUR GRAINS

While you reconsider your relationship with sugar, upgrade your approach to grains. Instead of simple grains like white flour, which your body processes in a way that's similar to how it handles sugars, consume more grains in whole form. Whole grains are cereal crops that contain a bran or outer shell. Think of the little crunchy bits in whole-grain bread. The bite and flavor come from the bran. This is how whole grains differ from refined grains, which are milled and stripped of their bran. White flour is typically refined this way.

"Refined grains, which lack the outer layer of the grain, lack a lot of beneficial nutrients," says Qi Sun, MD, ScD, MMS, assistant professor in the department of nutrition at Harvard's T.H. Chan School of Public Health. "Choosing to eat whole grains as one of the primary sources of carbohydrates in your diet is very critical," he says. "That would make a huge difference in terms of health consequences."

For one, whole grains contain fibers that can help you stay full and absorb carbohydrates more slowly. This way, your blood sugar will increase slowly in comparison with the quick spike you might have after eating refined grains, says Dr. Sun. What's more, according to the American Heart Association, the fiber often found in healthy whole grains helps the body fend off high cholesterol levels, heart disease, stroke, obesity, and type 2 diabetes. In fact, a 2013 study by the University of Leeds discovered that the risk of cardiovascular disease dropped dramatically for every 7 grams of fiber consumed.

Fiber is important, but it is far from the only star nutrient in whole grains. "The outer bran also contains polyphenols, including lignans and phenolic acid; minerals such as magnesium; and some B vitamins," says Dr. Sun. All of these nutrients have been linked to health benefits, including a reduced risk of diabetes, a precursor to heart disease. For maximum benefits, aim for three servings of whole grains per day by upgrading or adding the whole-grain foods we list here.

If whole grains aren't usually your jam, you can start slowly to get accustomed to their hearty taste and more complex texture. "In the beginning, you don't have to eat exclusively whole grains," said Dr. Sun. "You can blend whole grains with refined grains." Mix brown rice and white rice half and half, for instance. When you bake bread, use half white flour and half wheat flour. Gradually increase the ratio of whole grains to refined grains until you don't miss the refined ones anymore.

One more thing: Many people approach grains with caution because they fear gluten, which is present in wheat and some (but not all) other whole grains. A gluten-free diet is necessary if you have celiac disease or have been told by a doctor that you can't tolerate this protein. But, if your body *can* handle gluten, going for the gluten-free label might not be in your best interest. It turns out that gluten-free versions can contain more carbs and other less-than-desirable ingredients than the regular stuff.

"I wish people knew that gluten-free foods aren't all automatically healthy," Torey Armul, MS, RD, CSSD, LDN, spokesperson for the Academy of Nutrition and Dietetics, told us. "People often lose weight and feel better on a gluten-free diet, but it's usually not because of lack of gluten. It's because they're paying attention to their food choices and eating more real foods and less simple carbs. Gluten-free labeled packaged foods actually tend to have more calories and extra fat or sugar for added flavor."

Keep that in mind as you check out the following foods.

Amaranth

Amaranth is not technically a grain; rather, it's the seed of an amaranth plant that tastes like a whole grain and serves similar purposes. (Kind of like how tomatoes are fruits, but many people have trouble really thinking of them that way.) Amaranth is gluten-free, is packed with protein and fiber, and has a nutty-but-mild taste that will complement your greens.

Bread

Instead of white bread, buy bread with "whole grain" or "whole wheat" as the first ingredient. Ideally, the bread should have 1 gram of fiber for every 10 grams of carbohydrates. If the ingredients list has sugar, sucrose, corn syrup, or white or wheat flour near the top, skip it. Try a couple of our favorites, Ezekiel 4:9 Sprouted Whole Grain Bread and Nature's Own Double Fiber Wheat.

Crackers

Crunchy crackers are a uniquely satisfying snack, but the nutritional details on many popular crackers are less than satisfactory. We like Mary's Gone Crackers, which are made with whole grains and seeds instead of white flour. If you're going for nostalgia, try Reduced-Fat Triscuits, which are made with whole-grain wheat.

Kamut

Kamut, or Khorasan wheat, is a hearty ancient grain that deserves a spot on your plate. It's rich in heart-healthy omega-3 fatty acids, is high in protein (nearly 10 grams per cup!), and has a ton of heart-healthy fiber—21 grams per cup. A study in the *European Journal of Clinical Nutrition* found that participants who ate kamut wheat products in place of refined wheat reduced their total cholesterol, LDL cholesterol (the bad kind), and cytokines, which cause inflammation throughout the body, all in just eight weeks. Other grains that make great side dishes: freekeh and barley.

Noodles

The average American consumes 15.5 pounds of pasta each year—and most of it is made with the refined white stuff. This type of noodle is almost completely void of fiber and protein, two vital nutrients for weight loss. To boost the belly-filling fiber and hunger-busting protein in your meal, opt for a whole-grain noodle or a bean-based noodle. We like Banza Chickpea Shells and 365 Everyday Value Organic Whole Wheat Fusilli, for example. Another option? Put zucchini or other vegetables in a spiralizer to make veggie noodles. It's a fun way to hit your daily target of vegetable servings.

Oatmeal

Oatmeal isn't just a convenient morning meal; this whole grain may be one of the healthiest foods for your heart. A study review in the *British Journal of Nutrition* found that oatmeal reduces LDL ("bad" cholesterol), non-HDL cholesterol (total cholesterol minus the healthy cholesterol), and apolipoprotein B, which carries bad cholesterol through the body—all great news for your heart health. And at 4 grams of fiber per serving, oatmeal will keep you full until lunchtime if you do it right. To maximize satiety and prevent blood sugar spikes, add a little more fat and protein to your oatmeal. Stir in 1 tablespoon of nut butter or toss in some chia seeds or almond slivers. Don't skip a step and buy prepackaged flavored oatmeal. Some instant oatmeal packets contain as much as 14 grams of sugar. If you're on the go, Starbucks' Classic Whole-Grain Oatmeal is a great breakfast option, especially when you're on the go — but only if you just add the mixed nuts. Tossing in the brown sugar packet that comes with it adds in an additional 12 grams of sugar and 50 calories.

Popcorn

The soft crunch of popcorn is uniquely satisfying, and it can be a healthy pick, too. Plain popped corn is a healthy whole grain, but movie popcorn drenched in salt and fake butter is not. Invest in an air popper and skip the microwave bag. Multiple studies suggest that the chemicals that make those bags water repellent might harm your lungs.

Quinoa

This ancient seed has gained popularity in recent years for good reason. Cooked quinoa can stand alone as a side dish, and it also has surprising versatility. Add some to omelets. Coat chicken in it instead of breadcrumbs. Stir it into soups and chilis. Mix it into oats. Blend it into smoothies. Eating more quinoa could pay off. In a recent study published in *Current Developments in Nutrition*, people who were instructed to cook and consume 50 grams of quinoa (just under 1/3 cup) per day reduced their artery-clogging triglycerides and had fewer markers of metabolic syndrome by week 12 of the study.

Teff

This nutty-flavored gluten-free grain from Africa may be small, but it packs a mighty nutritional punch. It's loaded with fiber, essential amino acids, calcium, and vitamin C—a nutrient not typically found in grains. To reap the benefits, trade your morning oatmeal for a protein-packed teff porridge. Combine 1/2 cup of teff with a cup and a half of water and a pinch of salt in a medium saucepan. Let it come to a boil before reducing heat to low and letting it simmer for 15 to 20 minutes. Remove from heat and top with apples, cinnamon, and a dollop of natural peanut butter.

Tortillas

Tacos and burritos can be great components of a heart-healthy diet, so long as you stuff them with lots of vegetables, beans, and other good stuff instead of tons of sauces and other junk. Instead of white flour tortillas, pick up corn tortillas, whole-grain tortillas, or even some made with a nut flour, such as Siete Foods Almond Flour Tortillas.

Chapter 7 Action Summary

- Identify hidden sources of added sugars in your diet. (Read nutrition labels.)

- Replace sugary beverages with unsweetened tea, coffee, water, and other unsweetened drinks.

- Eat whole fruits instead of drinking fruit juices to benefit from the fruits' fiber.

- Ditch baked goods and other highly processed products made with refined white flour.

- Focus on whole grains.

8

Sleep 7 Hours or More Per Night

Your heart works better when your mind and body get enough rest.

WHEN YOU THINK about ways to live more healthfully, two things probably come to mind immediately: diet and exercise. You might not think about taking a nap. But scientific research continues to prove how vital sleep habits are to good health and, even, to weight loss.

When you sleep soundly, your blood pressure drops to its lowest point in the day, and if you don't get that refreshing break, then your BP can stay elevated, which may contribute to inflammation that gradually harms your blood vessels. In fact, people who say they sleep poorly are 14 percent more likely to have hypertension than people who don't, according to research published in the journal

Sleep Health. But it's not just your vessels that may suffer when you skimp on sleep. In a recent study published in the journal *Hypertension*, young adults who slept for only five hours for eight nights in a row had elevated heart rates compared to their normal rhythms. Over time, this could increase cardiovascular risk, the study authors say.

It's tempting to skimp on shut-eye, especially if you have kids, a busy job, aging parents to take care of, or any of the zillion responsibilities that keep us from hitting the pillow when we want to or ought to. That's why it's important to put sleep on a pedestal and plan your life around sleeping seven to nine hours per night. That's the sweet spot. But 35 percent of American adults fall short of the seven-hour mark, according to the Centers for Disease Control and Prevention.

"Contrary to the idea that most of us grew up with, sleep is not a waste of time," Christine M. Palumbo, MBA, RDN, FAND, told us. "In fact, it's a valuable use of your time and should be prioritized as part of your overall healthy lifestyle. Adequate amounts of quality sleep set the stage for good diet and exercise decisions during your waking hours."

If you have trouble falling asleep at night or you wake up feeling anything but refreshed, maybe a sleep disorder is interfering with your snoozing ability. About one in five American adults have insomnia, or trouble falling asleep, a study published in the journal *Sleep Medicine* suggests. If you have trouble falling asleep or staying asleep, a special type of therapy called cognitive behavioral therapy for insomnia, or CBT-I, could help you change your thoughts and behaviors in a way that will make sleep easier. In a study from Canada, people who received CBT-I started sleeping better, and 88 percent of them no longer had clinically significant insomnia by the end of the study.

Sleep restriction therapy, a component of CBT-I, helps you spend more time sleeping than trying to. Intrigued yet? The process begins with the patient logging the number of shut-eye hours they get per night for several weeks and then sticking to a consistent daily wake-up time. Once you've set your alarm clock to your desired time (and vowed not to hit snooze), make sure to hit the sack only when you're fully exhausted. If you actually sleep through the night until the alarm rings, you're encouraged to set a slightly earlier bedtime (about 15 minutes earlier than the night before) the next evening until you've clocked in your eight hours.

"By keeping patients awake for longer, we build up a strong sleep pressure," Matthew Walker, the director of the Sleep and Neuroimaging Lab at the University of California–Berkeley, wrote in his book, *Why We Sleep*. Instead of going to sleep when you think you're supposed to, hitting the pillow when you're too sleepy to keep your eyes open—no matter how long it takes—can help you delve into the deep, restful slumber you've been seeking. Doing so will also condition your mind to associate bed with sleep rather than the frustrating failure to achieve it. And while you may feel like a zombie the first few weeks of trying this method, you'll be thankful once you've cured chronic insomnia for good.

Meanwhile, between 3 and

FOOD FACT

32

Percentage of people with sleep issues who report being dissatisfied in their relationship, according to the National Sleep Foundation.

7 percent of adult men and 2 to 5 percent of adult women may have obstructive sleep apnea, a condition in which your airway becomes blocked at night, restricting your oxygen supply. Snoring is a common symptom, as is waking up gasping for air. Some people with sleep apnea don't notice anything at night; they simply feel tired and not refreshed during the day as a result of their poor sleep quality.

Heart disease and sleep apnea often go hand in hand, although it's not always clear whether the former causes the latter or vice versa. In a recent study from Italy, people with moderate or severe sleep apnea had more than triple the risk of a major heart attack or stroke than those without the same sleep trouble. If you're concerned that you may have sleep apnea, talk to your doctor. There are many treatments available, from oral appliances to machines that can help you breathe better at night.

For some people, a sleep disorder isn't the problem—stress is. In a study from New York University, people with emotional distress were 55 percent more likely to have unhealthy sleep. If worries, sadness, or other concerns interfere with your daily life, see a therapist. Our brains are complex machines that don't come with training manuals, and there's no shame in asking for help.

There are also some simple things you can do to reduce stress, improve sleep, and boost heart health all in one shot. For example, practice deep breathing. Slow, deliberate breathing fills your lungs with oxygen, decreasing the anxious feelings that often accompany being out of breath, and can slow a racing heart in the process. Researchers at the University of the Basque Country have even found that deep breathing exercises helped reduce levels of the stress hormone cortisol in both male and female study subjects.

Take a belly-expanding deep breath, hold it in for a few seconds, and then slowly exhale for five seconds. Repeat this pattern four times.

You might also benefit from a social media diet. Checking social media may make you feel connected to your friends and family even when you're far apart, but for many people, constantly checking these feeds increases stress. According to a study from the Pew Research Center, individuals who were exposed to stressful events via their friends' social media feeds were likely to internalize said stress. Put your phone away whenever possible and connect with the people in your life the old-fashioned way.

Another simple strategy is to put on your favorite tunes. Research published in *PLoS One* reveals that study subjects exposed to exterior stressors lowered their heart rate and salivary cortisol levels more quickly by listening to music than by listening to other supposedly relaxing sounds, such as running water.

No matter what's going on in your life, we want to help you develop healthy sleep habits.

Your Healthy Heart Diet Goal: Feel calmer and sleep soundly for seven to nine hours a night. These tips can help you snag more Z's.

Abandon your phone

Ask yourself, can this email wait until tomorrow? Then put the phone down before you hit the pillow. A study from the University of Haifa reveals that the blue light emitted from devices like smartphones can reduce the quantity and quality of your sleep. The reason: This light may suppress your body's production of melatonin, a sleep-inducing hormone. Put your phone away 20 minutes before your bedtime to avoid the light distraction. Read a book instead.

Coordinate with your spouse

Sync your sleep schedules, and resist the urge to watch one more episode of your latest Netflix binge while your partner hits the hay. Couples who sleep at the same times have lower blood pressure and lower levels of inflammation, according to research published in the journal *Sleep*. Sleeping next to a person you trust may help you balance stress hormones and other biological markers, the researchers say. Of course, there are exceptions. If your spouse snores loudly or has some other sleep problem that keeps you from sleeping soundly, encourage him or her to see a doctor about it, for both of your sakes.

Don't work out too late

Regular workouts have been found to help ease sleepless nights, but hitting the gym too late in the day can mess with your body clock. Exercising close to bedtime—within about two hours—can energize your body so much that it may not be able to wind down when it's time to call it a night. If you're not a morning person, try to exercise right after work or midday if your schedule allows. That way, you can head home, eat dinner, and relax knowing you'll be able to fall fast asleep when the time comes. If you're stuck at the office really late, you're better off skipping your workout for the night and hitting the hay early. If your body gets the rest it needs you're more likely to stay on track with your healthy eating and workouts in the days that follow.

Keep your pets out of your bed

We're not just talking about iguanas and boa constrictors. Don't let the dogs in for a cuddle. Or the cats. A study from the Mayo Clinic shows that having dogs in the bed reduced the amount and quality of sleep among study subjects. However, simply having them in the room was helpful—so consider investing in a mini bed fit for your furry prince or princess, and place it a few feet from yours.

Nighty Night Lights

Can't get to sleep? Turn the light on. But make sure it's one of these lights that are designed to help you establish a better sleep pattern. The Good Night bulb ($17) emits less of the blue light that suppresses production of the sleep hormone melatonin. The Drift Light ($30) is a self-dimming light that gradually dims to dark over 37 minutes, mimicking the setting sun.

Reconsider your midnight snack

A grumbling stomach could prevent you from falling asleep or wake you up mid-slumber, but eating too much too close to bedtime could leave you with acid reflux. If you're truly hungry, go with a light snack. Limit it to around 200 calories, and choose something substantial enough to keep hunger pangs at bay through the night but not so heavy that it will disrupt your sleep. Consider kiwi. In one study, participants who consumed two kiwifruits one hour before bedtime nightly for four weeks fell asleep 35 percent faster than those who didn't eat the New Zealand fruit. Besides being rich in antioxidants, carotenoids, and vitamins C and E, it also contains a familiar hormone, serotonin. This sleep hormone is related to rapid eye movement (REM) sleep, and low levels of it may cause insomnia. Similarly, kiwi is rich in folate, and insomnia is one of the health issues that are a symptom of folate deficiency. Also, skip chocolate at bedtime. Although dark chocolate is a heart-healthy snack, it should be a midday treat. The antioxidant-providing candy also contains caffeine, which can be a bump in the road for your body on its way to winding down.

Sip herbal tea

Many herbal teas offer sedative effects through their flavones, flavonoids, and resins. Passionflower tea has the flavone chrysin, which has antianxiety benefits and is a mild sedative, helping you calm nervousness so you can sleep at night. Another relaxing tea is lemon balm. A European study found that lemon balm serves as a natural sedative, and researchers reported that they observed reduced levels of sleep disorders among subjects using lemon balm versus those who were given a placebo. Valerian is another option. In a study of women, researchers gave half the test subjects a valerian extract and half a placebo. Up to 30 percent of those who received valerian reported an improvement in the quality of their sleep, versus just 4 percent of the control group. While scientists have yet to identify the exact active ingredient, they suspect that receptors in the brain may be stimulated to hit "sleep mode" when coming in contact with valerian.

Sleep in a dark, cold room

Exposure to light at night doesn't just interrupt your chances of a great night's sleep; it may also result in weight gain, according to a study published in the *American Journal of Epidemiology*. Study subjects who slept in the darkest rooms were 21 percent less likely to be obese than those sleeping in the lightest rooms. Meanwhile, not only do most people sleep better in a cooler temperatures, but our bodies respond more positively by activating more brown fat—the good fat that burns through the nasty, stubborn belly fat. A study published in the journal *Diabetes* found that people who switched to 66-degree sleeping temperatures doubled their good fat volumes.

Take a class in mindfulness meditation

Channeling your inner sense of peace and calm can help you snooze better. In a study published in *JAMA Internal Medicine*, older adults who took a two-hour mindfulness class once a week for six weeks improved their sleep quality. The researchers say meditation may promote relaxation and calm down the activity in brain areas that, when overactive, can keep you up at night. Channeling that inner "om" is the first step toward a more restful night in bed. Meditating or practicing other mindfulness exercises may help you achieve a feeling of calm that promotes restful sleep. In fact, research published in *JAMA Internal Medicine* reveals that mindfulness exercises significantly reduced sleep disturbances in a group of older adults. Meditation is also helpful for reducing anxiety, and a new study from Michigan Technology University suggests that even one session of meditation can reduce anxiety for up to a week and may also have blood pressure benefits. Sign me up!

Upgrade your bedding

Your mattress should be based on your weight (heavier people will need firmer mattresses) for proper back support, your pillow should support your neck, and your sheets should allow for proper temperature control. (Super-high thread counts—like 1,200—can sometimes make you sweaty because the fabric doesn't breathe.) Trust us: Once you make your bed the most comfortable place in your personal world, going to sleep will be all that easier.

Watch those nightcaps

A few glasses of wine might make you sleepy, but alcohol actually disrupts quality sleep in the long run. Research published in *Alcoholism: Clinical & Experimental Research* reveals that alcohol consumption reduces REM sleep, meaning you're less likely to wake up feeling refreshed in the morning. If you do choose to drink, make sure you have your last glass at least a few hours before bed, and follow it with plenty of water.

Chapter 8 Action Summary

- Try going to bed 15 minutes earlier tonight to see how you feel in the morning.

- Commit to a sleep schedule. Go to sleep at the same time each night and wake at the same time each morning—even on weekends.

- Practice good sleep hygiene.

- Avoid caffeine after 3 p.m.

- Reduce stress in your life and learn slumber-inducing strategies.

The 7-Day Healthy Heart Diet Meal Plan

Here's how to eat this week and for life!

FOR THE NEXT 7 days, follow our simple 6-step plan: Pile your plate with super heart foods; exercise every day; add healthy fats to meals; identify and destroy salt bombs; trim sugary carbs from your diet; and sleep seven hours or more per night. These steps are designed to help you lose weight, reduce several risk factors for heart disease, and just make you feel great! To hit all six steps of the plan, we recommend eating the following foods every day:

- 2 to 4 servings of fruits (about 1 cup or tennis ball–size portion each)

- 4 to 6 servings of vegetables (about 1 cup or fistful each)

- 3 servings of whole grains (about ½ cup of grains, which should fit in your cupped hand, or a slice of whole-grain bread)

- 2 servings of protein-rich lean meat, fish, dairy, or eggs (about 4 ounces of meat, which is the size of a deck of cards, or 8 ounces of dairy or one egg)

- 1 serving of nuts or seeds (about 1 ounce of whole nuts or seeds, 2 tablespoons or a Ping-Pong ball–size portion of nut or seed butter)

- 1 serving of legumes (about 1 cup of cooked beans)

What's more, if you avoid the added sugars and salt bombs we alerted you to earlier in this book, you will have a much easier time staying within the ideal ranges of **less than 1,500 to 2,300 milligrams** of salt per day and **under 6 teaspoons** of added sugar per day for women and **under 9 teaspoons** of added sugars per day for men. Every day of our meal plan delivers less than 2,300 milligrams of sodium, and many daily menus fall under 1,500 milligrams. Each day of suggested meals and snacks is also estimated to contain less than 6 teaspoons of added sugars. Again, check labels to make sure you aren't adding a processed food with more salt or sugar than you bargained for.

We've included a sample menu at the end of this chapter, along with a checklist to log your progress. Keep in mind that the servings outlined in the bulleted list above are not the only things you can eat. (You can pretty much always add more vegetables!) What's more, in our recipes in Chapter 10, we've pumped up these daily essentials with additional power foods and seasonings.

The point of this diet is not to be strict. We've designed it to be easy, delicious, and flexible. Feel free to mix up the sample menu with new fruits and vegetables, whole grains, or other heart-healthy options noted in the earlier chapters.

We aim for a calorie count between 1,500 and 1,700 calories per day to promote weight loss in women, but you might need to eat more if you are a man, work out strenuously, or fall within that lucky and small group of people who aren't carrying around excess weight. Remember, in this book we are writing for a broad audience, so we have to generalize our recommendations. For help determining exactly what you need given your health history, lifestyle, and unique circumstances, consult a registered dietitian nutritionist (with the letters RDN after their name). These professionals spend at least four years in college studying nutrition, plus close to 1,000 hours doing a supervised, hands-on internship, and they must pass an exam. With this much knowledge and experience in nutrition and the complexities of food science, they can really help you overhaul your diet.

Our diet plan focuses on whole foods, since foods are holistic packages of nutrients. However, it's smart to pay attention to the total count of carbs, fat, and protein you consume in a day. Scan the labels on your food, since nutritional contents vary. The Dietary Guidelines for Americans, which are assembled by a national panel of experts, recommend aiming for 45 to 65 percent of your daily calories from carbs, 20 to 35 percent from fats, and 10 to 35 percent from proteins. Every gram of carbs and protein is 4 calories, while every gram of fat is 9 calories. In a 1,600-calorie day, that means you should aim for about 180 to 260 grams of carbs, 35 to 62 grams of fat, and 40 to 140 grams of protein. Since many recent studies suggest that reducing carbs in favor of protein is favorable for weight loss, we aim to stay on the lower end of the carb range and the higher end of the protein range.

One of the best ways to follow our heart-healthy eating plan is to reduce your intake of processed and prepared foods and make more fresh foods at home. By preparing meals at home, you can maintain control over what you take in, which makes it easier to keep your intake of calories, added sugars, and sodium within healthy limits. Our recipes, beginning on page 163, are designed to be simple, but brushing up on a few cooking skills can't hurt. Here are a few good tips:

- **Broil.** The broiler is really nothing more than an inverted grill; a source of concentrated, quick-cooking heat. Since most broilers have only two settings—on or off—they're really easy to use. Just set the oven to broil and let it heat up for about 5 minutes before you start cooking your food. Thin cuts of chicken, pork chops, steaks, and fresh vegetables take about 10 minutes to broil; just be sure to flip them midway through the process so they're evenly cooked.

- **Assemble a salad.** Master the art of making a few basic salads. A basic house salad contains spinach, onion, tomatoes, carrots, and bell pepper; a classic Greek salad is filled with things like romaine, onion, olives, bell peppers, tomatoes, cucumber, and feta cheese. Pair either salad with a slice of Ezekiel bread or some grilled fish or chicken to turn it into a full-on entrée!

- **Adapt recipes.** Every good cook knows that recipe ingredients don't have to be set in stone. Mushrooms can stand in for eggplant, and pricey ingredients you don't think you'll ever use again can often be omitted. If you understand what tastes good together, the possibilities for tasty creations is infinite.

- **Tenderize chicken.** Thicker cuts of boneless chicken are more affordable than the thin-cut kind. Thankfully, if you have a chicken tenderizer, you can flatten out thick chicken cuts to make them just as tender, moist, and easy to cook with as their skinny counterparts. Before you start pounding away at the meat, though, you'll need to cover it with a piece of plastic wrap or put it into a plastic zip-locking bag. This will prevent small pieces of meat and meat juices from getting all over your counter. Once you're prepped and ready to roll, go back and forth over the meat using a hammering motion with the tenderizer until the meat reaches the desired thickness.

- **Scramble eggs.** After you've cracked your eggs into a bowl and beaten them with a whisk or a fork, pour the mixture into a warm, oiled frying pan, and scatter your fillings. We like to add things like chopped veggies and herbs. Once the egg begins to solidify, fold it in half. When it's no longer runny, it's time to eat.

- **Roast veggies.** Roasted vegetables are one of the most deliciously savory—and not to mention, easy and versatile—dishes around. You can make them in bulk and add them to salads, egg dishes, and wraps or simply heat 'em up and pair them with a whole grain and a protein. To pull together the dish, chop up your favorite roasting veggies (we like carrots, onions, broccoli, brussels sprouts, and sweet potatoes) and lay them out on a foil-wrapped sheet pan. Next, drizzle with some extra-virgin olive oil and dried herbs and spices (garlic powder, rosemary, ground pepper, and oregano are good), and toss them into a 400°F oven for about 40 minutes, or until the veggies are tender. That's it!

- **Make simple soups.** It's what you slurp when you're sick, cold, or just in the mood to get into the fall spirit. Yes, that's right, we're talking about soup. Sure, you could grab a can opener and choke down the canned variety, but we think you deserve better than that. Making a soup from scratch isn't rocket science; most don't even require recipes. You can easily just toss some chopped veggies, canned beans, and cooked cubed chicken into a simmering pot of low-sodium chicken broth and call it a day.

We also know that there's a good chance you'll end up at a restaurant or two in the next 7 to 14 days, so check our favorite picks and advice for navigating that on page 217. And since products vary, the nutritional details may shake out a little bit differently in practice. One way to increase the chances that you'll hit the right marks? Make sure that your plate is half full of fruits and vegetables at every meal, that you eat more whole grains than refined grains, and that each meal has a source of healthy protein and fat.

Every day of our plan features three meals and one snack. We've included a snack a day in our meal plan because we know that hunger pangs happen. If you're truly hungry, then a snack is in order; however, if you find that you munch mindlessly throughout the day, it's time to rethink your habits. Nutrition experts are starting to question the value of snacking because it's so difficult to enjoy snacks in moderation. Consider the results of this study published recently in the journal *Obesity*: More than 360 overweight people were supervised in following a highly restrictive diet for 24 months. The researchers monitored the subjects' body weights and craving levels periodically and found that their cravings for certain foods decreased only when the frequency with which they ate those foods decreased, not when they simply ate less of the foods. The scientists from Pennington Biomedical Research Center who conducted the experiment say it suggests that if you're trying to lose weight and you usually have strong craving for chocolate, you'll be more successful at curbing those cravings if you avoid chocolate altogether.

"The more I see the research, the more I'm getting away from snacking," says Judy Caplan, MS, RDN, author of *GoBeFull*. Every time you eat, your body has an insulin response, and you don't want too many of these metabolic responses per day because, over time, your insulin sensitivity can decrease, which is an early step toward type 2 diabetes. If you do need a snack, pick something balanced. Take cues from Caplan: "If I were going to eat a snack, I might take a big leaf of romaine and roll up some nitrite-free turkey breast with an asparagus spear and a red pepper, or I might grab a handful of nuts," she says. "Maybe I would do celery and natural peanut butter."

In general, it's important to eat when you are hungry and not haphazardly. The American Heart Association reports that the way you time your meals matters to your heart. Here's why: Your body operates under a central clock that is encoded into your brain and some of your organs.

Your sleep patterns and light exposure play major roles in setting and maintaining this clock, but your diet can shift it, too. Your liver's internal clock may be especially perturbed by erratic meal timing, and that's a problem because your liver is involved in the production of artery-clogging lipids. For example, a 2017 study from the University of Pennsylvania School of Medicine showed that people who waited until around 11 p.m. for their last bites of food had higher cholesterol and triglycerides, markers of an increased risk of heart problems.

THE HEALTHY HEART DIET SAMPLE MENU

Following are 14 days of various healthy meal combinations. Why fourteen menus for a 7-day plan? Well, you're not going to stop eating after 7 days, are you? We wanted to show you how much flexibility you have when planning heart-healthy meals. Enjoy! Bonus points if you can add even more vegetables to the mix! (Note: If your calorie needs are higher, simply add carefully considered portions of the super heart foods outlined earlier in the book.)

Day 1

Breakfast: Very Berry Yogurt Bowl (recipe on page 164) and a slice of whole-grain toast with 1 Tbsp nut butter

Lunch: Spicy Red Lentils with Cauliflower (recipe on page 169) and 1 cup of air-popped popcorn with 1 tsp olive oil and 1 tsp salt

Dinner: Roasted Chicken, Vegetables, and Quinoa (recipe on page 174)

Snack: Large banana with 1 Tbsp almond butter

Day 1 nutrition total:
1,573 calories, 60 g fat, 986 mg sodium, 192 g carbs, 36 g fiber, 72 g protein

Day 2

Breakfast: Breakfast Burrito (recipe on page 163) and a sliced beefsteak tomato

Lunch: Leftover Spicy Red Lentils with Cauliflower and an apple

Dinner: Chicken Salad Sandwich with Curry and Raisins (recipe on page 175) and a navel orange

Snack: 1 cup jicama slices and 2 Tbsp nut butter

Day 1 nutrition total:
1,605 calories, 64 g fat, 2,170 mg sodium, 190 g carbs, 32 g fiber, 71 g protein

---

Day 3

Breakfast: Grapefruit, ½ ounce pistachios, and 1 packet instant steel-cut oatmeal

Lunch: Avocado, Tomato, Corn, and Salmon Salad with Cilantro-Lime Dressing (recipe on page 168)

Dinner: Pork Fried Rice (recipe on page 178; make 1 extra cup brown rice) and Asian Slaw (recipe on page 179)

Snack: Chocolate-Covered Strawberries (recipe on page 192) and five regular strawberries

Day 1 nutrition total:
1,642 calories, 62 g fat, 1,449 mg sodium, 214 g carbs, 29 g fiber, 79 g protein

Day 4

Breakfast: Banana Bread Mug Muffin (recipe on page 164) and a hard-boiled egg

Lunch: Leftover Pork Fried Rice

Dinner: Creamy Tomato Basil Soup (recipe on page 180) and a slice of whole-grain toast

Snack: Awesome Guacamole (recipe on page 193) with 1 cup celery sticks

Day 1 nutrition total:
1,553 calories, 55 g fat, 1,619 mg sodium, 206 g carbs, 36.5 g fiber, 75 g protein

Day 5

Breakfast: Tofu Scramble and Toast (recipe on page 165; add an extra ½ cup spinach) and an apple

Lunch: Chinese Chicken Salad (recipe on page 170) and a large fresh navel orange

Dinner: Turkey Burger Mediterranean Style (recipe on page 181), Baked Sweet Potato Fries (recipe on page 182), and Sweet and Sour Onions (recipe on page 183)

Snack: 1 cup grapes and ¼ cup almonds

Day 1 nutrition total:
1,574 calories, 61 g fat, 1,346 mg sodium, 190 g carbs, 30 g fiber, 85 g protein

Day 6

Breakfast: Spicy Avocado Toast with Fried Egg and Tomato (recipe on page 166), 1 extra piece of toast, and a cup of blueberries

Lunch: Leftover Chinese Chicken Salad and a large fresh navel orange

Dinner: Chicken Fajitas (recipe on page 184)

Snack: Hummus with Celery and Cucumbers (recipe on page 194) plus a large apple

Day 6 nutrition total:
1,673 calories, 68 g fat, 1,363 mg sodium, 188 g carbs, 25.5 g fiber, 98 g protein

Day 7

Breakfast: Banana Chocolate Chip Breakfast Quesadilla (recipe on page 166) and 8 oz plain kefir

Lunch: Chicken Portobello Wrap (recipe on page 171)

Dinner: Pumpkin Turkey Chili (recipe on page 185), ½ cup brown rice, and the other half of the banana from breakfast

Snack: ¼ cup almonds, 1 cup Bing cherries

Day 7 nutrition total:
1,677 calories, 55 g fat, 1,023 mg sodium, 191 g carbs, 25 g fiber, 110 g protein

MORE MENUS

Day 8

Breakfast: Peaches and Cream Yogurt Parfait (recipe on page 167)

Lunch: Leftover Pumpkin Turkey Chili and ½ cup brown rice

Dinner: Fettuccine with Chicken with Roasted Vegetables (recipe on page 186)

Snack: Awesome Guacamole (recipe on page 193) with 1 cup celery sticks

Day 8 nutrition total:
1,641 calories, 46 g fat, 1,086 mg sodium, 235 g carbs, 45 g fiber, 99 g protein

Day 9

Breakfast: Ricotta Toast (recipe on page 167)

Lunch: 2 servings of Minestrone with Pesto (recipe on page 172)

Dinner: Shrimp Fajitas (recipe on page 187) and ½ cup fresh pineapple

Snack: 2 Low-FODMAP Snack Balls (recipe on page 195)

Day 9 nutrition total:
1,577 calories, 56 g fat, 215 g carbs, 1,715 mg added sodium, 59 g fiber, 94 g protein

Day 10

Breakfast: Banana Bread Mug Muffin (recipe on page 164) and a hard-boiled egg

Lunch: 2 leftover servings of Minestrone with Pesto

Dinner: San Antonio Rice Bowl (recipe on page 186) plus an extra ¼ cup instant brown rice and a large apple

Snack: 1 cup grapes and ¼ cup almonds

Day 10 nutrition total:
1,560 calories, 56 g fat, 223 g carbs, 61 g fiber, 82 g protein

Day 11

Breakfast: Tofu Scramble and Toast (recipe on page 165; add an extra ½ cup of spinach) plus an apple

Lunch: Chicken Salad Sandwich with Curry and Raisins (recipe on page 175) plus a navel orange

Dinner: Cedar Plank Salmon (recipe on page 189) and Roasted Parmesan Asparagus (recipe on page 190)

Snack: 1 cup of jicama slices and 2 Tbsp nut butter

Day 11 nutrition total:
1,600 calories, 56 g fat, 1,287 mg sodium, 173 g carbs, 62.4 g fiber without asparagus, 99 g protein

Day 12

Breakfast: Very Berry Yogurt Bowl (recipe on page 164) plus a slice of whole-grain toast with 1 Tbsp peanut butter

Lunch: Spicy Red Lentils with Cauliflower (recipe on page 169) and 1 cup of air-popped popcorn with 1 tsp olive oil and 1 tsp salt

Dinner: Roasted Chicken, Vegetables, and Quinoa (recipe on page 174)

Snack: Large banana with 1 Tbsp almond butter

Day 12 nutrition total:
1,573 calories, 60 g fat, 986 mg sodium, 192 g carbs, 1.5 tsp added sugars, 42 g fiber, 72 g protein

Day 13

Breakfast: Peaches and Cream Yogurt Parfait (recipe on page 167)

Lunch: Pumpkin Turkey Chili (recipe on page 185) and ½ cup brown rice

Dinner: Fettuccine with Chicken and Roasted Vegetables (recipe on page 186)

Snack: Awesome Guacamole (recipe on page 193) with 1 cup celery sticks

Day 13 nutrition total:
1,641 calories, 46 g fat, 1,086 mg sodium, 235 g carbs, 46 g fiber, 99 g protein

Day 14

Breakfast: Lemon Kale Protein Detox (recipe on page 173) plus ⅛ cup almonds

Lunch: Grilled cheese sandwich made with two slices whole-grain bread and 2 oz Swiss cheese, plus a large apple

Dinner: Baked Halibut (recipe on page 191) and 1 cup cooked quinoa

Snack: Hummus with Celery and Cucumbers (recipe on page 194) plus a large sliced bell pepper

Day 14 nutrition total:
1,529 calories, 60 g fat, 928 mg sodium, 150 g carbs, 59 g fiber without almonds, 102 g protein

Your Diet Checklist

Keep tabs on your daily servings on this checklist and notice where you have room for improvement. For example, if you are struggling to make your vegetable mark, stock up on precut and frozen veggies at the grocery store so you can make them in a snap. If whole grains are a problem, make a large batch in a rice cooker and freeze pre-portioned containers. This checklist is good for 14 days. Make copies if you need more.

Day 1

- **Fruits** _____

- **Vegetables** _____

- **Whole grains** _____

- **Protein-rich meat, eggs, fish, or dairy** _____

- **Nuts/seeds** _____

- **Legumes** _____

Day 2

- **Fruits** _____
- **Vegetables** _____
- **Whole grains** _____
- **Protein-rich meat, eggs, fish, or dairy** _____
- **Nuts/seeds** _____
- **Legumes** _____

Day 3

- **Fruits** _____
- **Vegetables** _____
- **Whole grains** _____
- **Protein-rich meat, eggs, fish, or dairy** _____
- **Nuts/seeds** _____
- **Legumes** _____

Day 4

- **Fruits** _____
- **Vegetables** _____
- **Whole grains** _____
- **Protein-rich meat, eggs, fish, or dairy** _____
- **Nuts/seeds** _____
- **Legumes** _____

Day 5

- **Fruits** _____
- **Vegetables** _____
- **Whole grains** _____
- **Protein-rich meat, eggs, fish, or dairy** _____
- **Nuts/seeds** _____
- **Legumes** _____

Day 6

- **Fruits** _____

- **Vegetables** _____

- **Whole grains** _____

- **Protein-rich meat, eggs, fish, or dairy** _____

- **Nuts/seeds** _____

- **Legumes** _____

Day 7

- **Fruits** _____

- **Vegetables** _____

- **Whole grains** _____

- **Protein-rich meat, eggs, fish, or dairy** _____

- **Nuts/seeds** _____

- **Legumes** _____

Day 8

- **Fruits** _____
- **Vegetables** _____
- **Whole grains** _____
- **Protein-rich meat, eggs, fish, or dairy** _____
- **Nuts/seeds** _____
- **Legumes** _____

Day 9

- **Fruits** _____
- **Vegetables** _____
- **Whole grains** _____
- **Protein-rich meat, eggs, fish, or dairy** _____
- **Nuts/seeds** _____
- **Legumes** _____

Day 10

- Fruits _____

- Vegetables _____

- Whole grains _____

- Protein-rich meat, eggs, fish, or dairy _____

- Nuts/seeds _____

- Legumes _____

Day 11

- Fruits _____

- Vegetables _____

- Whole grains _____

- Protein-rich meat, eggs, fish, or dairy _____

- Nuts/seeds _____

- Legumes _____

Day 12

- Fruits _____

- Vegetables _____

- Whole grains _____

- Protein-rich meat, eggs, fish, or dairy _____

- Nuts/seeds _____

- Legumes _____

Day 13

- Fruits _____

- Vegetables _____

- Whole grains _____

- Protein-rich meat, eggs, fish, or dairy _____

- Nuts/seeds _____

- Legumes _____

Day 14

- **Fruits** _____

- **Vegetables** _____

- **Whole grains** _____

- **Protein-rich meat, eggs, fish, or dairy** _____

- **Nuts/seeds** _____

- **Legumes** _____

SIMPLE WAYS TO COOK ONCE AND EAT ALL WEEK

For some people, cooking every day is not an option, and that's when Sunday meal prep can be life-changing. Whether you cook full recipes or just prepare a few healthy basics for a meal-prep buffet, stocking your fridge with the right kinds of fuel will save you time—and calories—throughout the week. With a little know-how and planning, you can easily prep 7 days' worth of meals and snacks over the weekend, ensuring your diet doesn't fall off track during the hectic workweek. To help you strategize, we compiled some of the best Sunday meal prep tips to help you get out of those mid- and late-week takeout ruts.

Buy in bulk

Because you'll be prepping for the whole week, it makes sense to purchase most of your items in bulk not only to have enough but also to save money! Boneless chicken breasts, one of the priciest cuts of poultry, is only $33.73 at Costco for a 9.14-pound pack, but would ring out to $40.41 at a local supermarket.

Check your schedule

You have to do more than plan *what* you're going to eat for the week; it's also important to plan *when* you'll eat your healthy meals. Do you need breakfast, lunch, and dinner every day, or is there an office meeting with a team lunch on Monday? Are you going on a business trip on Thursday? Are your parents coming to visit? Maybe you planned to meet up with a friend one night. Make sure to factor in exactly how many days you need to be prepping for.

Cook small

Instead of making large casserole-style dishes, if you're making something like meatloaf, make it in individual portions instead of as a whole loaf. Or, choose recipes like muffins that are already made pre-portioned. That way, when you freeze it, it will thaw quickly and you'll be ready to go!

Create building blocks

Similar to a bouillon cube, you can make yourself meal building blocks to get dinner started in a jiffy. Freeze pre-portioned packets of chicken or vegetable stock, pesto, or herb compound butter, or make up baggies of your own spice mixes—oregano, basil, parsley, and thyme for an

Italian dish; onion, garlic, and chili powder, paprika, cumin, and cayenne pepper for a fajita seasoning; and chili powder, cumin, coriander, cayenne, paprika, and garlic powder for any barbeque rub.

Double up

If you want to make full recipes to eat throughout the week, pick recipes that make large batches or choose ones that you can double. Even if a recipe is intended for one person or one night, just doubling or tripling it will allow you to cook once and eat for a week. Before you head to the store, do the calculations. Usually, the rule of thumb is to double big items like fats, proteins, and produce, but adjust smaller items like spices and seasonings to taste. And when it comes to cooking, it usually won't be double the time. Check the recipe for doneness at the time called for in the recipe, and if it's not ready, check again in roughly five-minute increments.

Find ingredient overlaps

When picking recipes for meal prep, try grouping them by overlapping ingredients. If you need to make rice one night for a chicken curry dish, you can use it later in the week for fried rice. Spinach can be used in a salad or in the filling of lasagna roll-ups.

Get proper containers

Mason jars, Tupperware, and plastic bags will all do. You can also check out a local restaurant-supply shop for some takeout-style containers. If you're unhappy with your plastic containers, recycle them and replace them with stainless steel or glass containers. If you're going to go plastic, choose BPA-free containers with lockable lids to prevent spilling.

Get your grains

Whole-wheat pastas, quinoa, farro, rice, barley...whatever your pick, get your grain on. These grains can be used as sides, as the base of a bowl, or in main dishes like fried rice. Usually, these grains will last in the fridge for two to three days, so be sure to freeze a portion if you plan to eat it later in the week.

Go raw

Fully cooking batches of casseroles, soups, enchiladas, or pasta dishes that you can reheat in the microwave or oven are always great, but "despite what many people think, you don't have to cook entire meals ahead of time—that can be overwhelming" Stephanie Brookshier, RDN, ACSM-CPT, assured us. Instead of baking, just prep all your food on Sunday and sequester it raw into baggies. This way, you don't feel like you're eating leftovers every day. You can throw a bag of pre-portioned chicken and veggies into the slow cooker before work or put an unbaked, frozen casserole dish in the oven right when you get home. Sometimes, just a little shortcut here and there will save you hours in the long run.

Ice it right

Not all food will last the whole week in the fridge, so be sure to freeze some of it. After you've cooked your food, you have to make sure it cools completely before putting it in the freezer. When you put away food while it's still warm, it can raise the general temperature of the freezer. When this happens, the food around the warmer addition may partially thaw and refreeze, which alters its taste and texture. Moisture can also evaporate and condense in the plastic container, which will make its contents mushy. To keep food safe, cool freshly cooked dishes by placing the food in a wide, shallow container and refrigerate, uncovered, until cool. With soups, you can pour them into a metal bowl and set the bowl in an ice bath.

Label, label, label

Use dry-erase markers for plastic and glass containers, or use a Sharpie on a piece of tape or directly on a plastic bag. If you're making individual, pre-portioned meals, use a particular color Sharpie to designate the day of the week a meal corresponds to. If you're freezing food, be sure to label it with the date you made it or its date of expiration. Food will usually last three months in a freezer, but that guideline is for quality only. Safety-wise, frozen foods should be OK indefinitely.

Master your freezer

Some foods are better suited to freezing and reheating than others: "Soups, broths, smoothies, and sauces can be frozen in ice cube trays, which comes in handy for portion control and weight management. Veggie-based casseroles, whole-grain-wrap burritos, and homemade turkey or veggie burgers can be frozen individually, giving family members a healthy grab-and-go option," Stephanie Brookshier, RDN, ACSM-CPT told us. When your meal is already made and only needs to be reheated, you're less likely to give into calling for takeout on hectic evenings.

Mix things up

If you can't fathom eating the same thing two days in a row, plan on making two or three different dishes that you can alternate or mix and match throughout the week. With the right planning and creativity, you can make the same food go a long way. By just making different sauces, prepped chicken and vegetables can be used to make a quick stir-fry one night, fajitas the next, and a salad or pasta dish the following night.

Optimize freezer storage

Use moisture-proof zip-locking bags and containers to help minimize freezer burn. Store foods in small servings to help them freeze quickly and to allow you to defrost only what you need. If you're storing individual servings of something like pancakes, freeze everything first in a single layer. Then stuff them all into a bag so they won't stick together. For soups and stews, keep them in a plastic bag to save space: Fill the bag and flatten it as you seal it to remove air and allow it to be stackable.

Organize your fridge

With all this prepped food, you're going to need some fridge space. Put the foods that will be used earliest in the week in the front and foods for the end of the week toward the back. Be sure to clean out your fridge weekly to keep food fresh. To increase the shelf life of your produce, separate ethylene producers—foods like avocados, ripe bananas, and tomatoes, which release this naturally occurring plant hormone that speeds up their ripening process—from the veggies that are spoiled by the gas (broccoli, spinach, and sweet potatoes, for instance).

Prep your protein

If you're happy using more of a buffet-style meal prep, be sure to prep one or two proteins, such as chicken, black beans, or eggs. You can keep them in the fridge to use in wraps, salads, sandwiches, or Buddha bowls. If you're making chicken, consider buying a ready-made rotisserie chicken or roasting your own! This will help cut down on individual cooking times. Meat proteins can be kept in the fridge from three to four days.

Print a plan

To keep on top of everything, print out a meal schedule so you know which meal was planned for which day, and when. Set a notification on your phone to remind you that you'll have to defrost something one day to be used the next.

Start chopping

Wash, chop, and prepare most of your veggies for the week—whether they're going to be left raw or used in a cooked dish—and store them in Tupperware containers. Ilyse Schapiro, MS, RD, told us: "I love vegetables, but I'm more likely to eat and cook them if they're cut and ready to go. Store each vegetable in an individual container so when it comes time to cook, all you have to do is grab the ones you want and get to work. They're also great to have on hand to snack on when you get hungry." There are a few exceptions, though. For example, slicing strawberries ahead of time is a mistake because oxidation devalues some of their nutrition, and an herb like mint is best chopped immediately before you use it.

Utilize your gadgets

It's not easy to make two or three dishes by yourself. Why not break out those unused wedding gifts? Slow cookers, rice cookers, pressure cookers, microwaves, toaster ovens, air fryers? Utilize them all! Yes, it might mean for a little extra cleanup, but it will drastically cut down on your prep time.

Bon appétit! Now for the easy part! You've prepped and cooked your meals, so all you have to do is pack them in a bag to ensure a day of healthy eating. If you've frozen food, defrost it in the refrigerator—roughly five hours per pound—or in the microwave.

Chapter 9 Action Summary

- Use meal planning to keep your diet on track.

- Cook more, go out to eat less.

- Prepare some meals and snacks on Sunday for use during the week to make cooking quicker and less stressful.

- Use your diet checklist to ensure that you are getting the required amounts and varieties of foods recommended for healthy heart nutrition.

10

The Healthy Heart Recipes

A selection of delicious recipes featuring superfoods that show you how easy it is to eat for good cardiovascular health.

HE RECIPES that follow complement the Healthy Heart Diet sample menus starting on page 137. We hope you also add them to your permanent rotation of favorite dishes. Each recipe in this chapter boasts one or more of the heart-healthy ingredients we've identified in this book, from super heart foods to whole grains to nuts.

What's more, these dishes all taste great. We aren't serving up bland recipes devoid of flavor. The reality is that it's pretty tough to stick to a diet if you don't enjoy eating the food. That's why we've taken foods you already love, from burritos to tomato soup, and made them healthier.

We've even created a slimmed-down version of a burger with fries. We've got muffins, parfaits, and more to satisfy your sweet tooth.

In these recipes, the ingredients are combined to give you a variety of tasty experiences, from savory to sweet to sour to spicy. Some recipes contain small amounts of salt and sugar to enhance their flavor without going into the danger zone. We, of course, recommend going easy when directed to add "salt and pepper, to taste." Always taste before you add more, sticking to the plan to reduce added salt in your foods.

We also have taken care to include ingredients that won't cost a fortune and are easily available. Best of all, these recipes are flexible. If you want to add even more fruits and vegetables, have at it! If you want to substitute one heart-healthy ingredient for another, go for it! Sure, you can put orange slices in the Very Berry Yogurt Bowl if you don't have berries on hand. *Of course* you can add broccoli to the Roasted Chicken, Vegetables, and Quinoa recipe if brussels sprouts aren't your veg of choice.

Cooking (and eating) can be healthy and fun activities at the same time. For more inspiration, check out our recipes page at eatthis.com. And for even more heart-healthy recipes, visit the American Heart Association's recipes page at recipes.heart.org.

BREAKFAST RECIPES

Breakfast Burrito

What you'll need

1   egg scrambled in your choice of cooking oil or spray
¼   avocado, sliced
1   medium 8" (soft-taco-size) whole-grain tortilla
Shredded cheddar cheese
Salsa
Salt and pepper, to taste

How to make it

Scramble eggs and place in the middle of the tortilla. Immediately top with shredded cheese so the heat of the eggs melts it. Add sliced avocado and salsa. Fold in the sides, then the bottom of the tortilla, and then roll the burrito up to the top.

Makes 1 serving

Per serving: 303 calories, 15 g fat (5 g saturated), 882 mg sodium, 24 g carbs, 7 g fiber, 12 g protein

Very Berry Yogurt Bowl

What you'll need

1	cup plain Greek yogurt
½	cup mixed berries (strawberries, blueberries, blackberries, raspberries)
1	tsp lemon juice and lemon rind
1	Tbsp mint, chopped
1	tsp honey

How to make it

Mix yogurt, lemon juice, lemon rind, and honey in a bowl. Top with berries and fresh mint.

Makes 1 serving

Per serving: 289 calories, 11 g fat (8 g saturated), 94 mg sodium, 16 g carbs, 4 g fiber, 24 g protein

---

Banana Bread Mug Muffin

What you'll need

¼	cup rolled oats
2	Tbsp vanilla almond milk
1	tsp maple syrup
1	egg
1	banana, mashed

Pinch of salt

How to make it

Whisk together milk, honey, salt, and egg. Add your oats and mashed banana, and stir until combined. Pop in the microwave for 2 minutes, checking the mug after every 30 seconds and waiting 10 seconds before putting it back in.

Makes 1 serving

Per serving: 280 calories, 7 g fat (2 g saturated), 104 mg sodium, 47 g carbs, 5 g fiber, 10 g protein

Tofu Scramble and Toast

Even the most devoted carnivore can benefit from the occasional vegan meal, and breakfast is a great place to start.

What you'll need

½   cup firm tofu

1   cup spinach

Turmeric, to taste

¼   cup Bob's Red Mill Large Flake Nutritional Yeast

1   slice Ezekiel Sprouted Whole Grain Bread

How to make it

Sauté the firm tofu and spinach and mix in a sprinkle of turmeric and the Bob's Red Mill Large Flake Nutritional Yeast for flavor and protein. Serve over a slice of toasted Ezekiel Sprouted Whole Grain Bread for some high-quality carbohydrates and fiber.

Makes 1 serving

Per serving: 255 calories, 8 g fat (1 g saturated), 156 mg sodium, 34 g carbs, 9 g fiber, 21 g protein

Spicy Avocado Toast with Fried Egg and Tomato

What you'll need

1   slice whole wheat toast
1   egg
½   avocado
Paprika, to taste
Salt and pepper, to taste
2   slices of tomato
Dash of hot sauce

How to make it

While the bread is toasting, fry an egg in a nonstick pan. Mash half an avocado directly on the toast, and sprinkle with paprika, salt, and pepper. Layer on two slices of tomato and top with your egg. Finish with hot sauce.

Makes 1 serving

Per serving: 263 calories, 16 g fat, 415 mg sodium, 20 g carbs, 7 g fiber, 11 g protein

Banana Chocolate Chip Breakfast Quesadilla

What you'll need

1   whole grain tortilla (we like Food for Life Ezekiel 4:9 Sprouted Whole Grain Tortilla)
1   Tbsp peanut butter (we like Adam's Creamy Peanut Butter)
½   medium banana, sliced
1   heaping Tbsp dark chocolate chips

How to make it

Spread peanut butter over tortilla, place tortilla in a large non-stick skillet. Add sliced banana to half the tortilla. Sprinkle the same half of the tortilla with chocolate chips. Fold tortilla over fillings. Heat on medium until chocolate melts and tortilla becomes crisp. Slice and serve.

Makes 1 serving

Per serving: 366 calories, 16 g fat, 203 mg sodium, 50 g carbs, 9 g fiber, 11 g protein

Peaches and Cream Yogurt Parfait

What you'll need

1	cup yogurt (ideally plain Greek yogurt)
1	Tbsp grated ginger
1	Tbsp honey
1	sliced peach
1	Tbsp flaxseeds

How to make it

Grate fresh ginger into a cup of yogurt with honey, stir to combine. Top with peach slices and flaxseeds.

Makes 1 serving

Per serving: 314 calories, 8 g fat, 4 mg sodium, 35 g carbs, 6 g fiber, 26 g protein

Ricotta Toast

What you'll need

½	cup Polly-O part-skim ricotta cheese
2	slices Ezekiel Sprouted Whole Grain Bread
1	teaspoon honey
½	cup blackberries

How to make it

Spread the ricotta on top of two toasted slices of the bread and drizzle with the honey for a touch of sweetness. Top with the blackberries to up your antioxidant intake for the day.

Makes 1 serving

Per serving: 392 calories, 13 g fat, 281 mg sodium, 47 g carbs, 16 g fiber, 25 g protein

LUNCH RECIPES

Avocado, Tomato, Corn, and Salmon Salad with Cilantro-Lime Dressing

What you'll need

Cooked salmon fillet
¼   avocado
½   tomato
Handful of frozen corn
2   cups lettuce (we like romaine)
1   cup cilantro
1   clove garlic
Juice of 1 lime
Salt and pepper, to taste
2   Tbsp white vinegar
3   Tbsp extra-virgin olive oil

How to make it

Combine the first five ingredients to make the salad. In a separate container, combine the last six ingredients to make the dressing. Drizzle half the dressing over the salad, and save the other half for another day.

Makes 1 serving of salad, 2 servings of dressing

Per 1 dressed salad: 489 calories, 29 g fat, 422 mg sodium, 33 g carbs, 9 g fiber, 31 g protein

Spicy Red Lentils with Cauliflower

Recipe by Erin Peisach

What you'll need

½   cup dry red lentils
2   Tbsp extra-virgin olive oil
1   small onion, chopped
2   tsp minced garlic
2½ cups water
1¼ tsp ground cumin
2   tsp curry powder
¼   tsp turmeric
½   tsp sea salt
2   cups chopped raw cauliflower
½   tsp minced ginger
½   lemon, juiced
1   Tbsp tomato paste
¼   tsp cayenne pepper
¼   cup chopped cilantro

How to make it

- In a large saucepan over medium heat, add 1 tablespoon of oil. Then toss in the onion and garlic and sauté for 5 to 7 minutes.

- Add in the red lentils, spices (cumin, curry powder, turmeric, salt), and 2 cups of water. Bring the mixture to a boil, and then drop to a low simmer and cover for 25 to 30 minutes.

- Meanwhile in a separate pan, add 1 tablespoon of oil to medium heat. Then toss in the cauliflower, ginger, lemon juice, tomato paste, and cayenne pepper. Add ½ cup of water. Mix all the ingredients together and allow them to cook for 10 to 12 minutes.

- Combine the cooked cauliflower to the cooked red lentils. Mix until well combined. Finally, turn off the heat and mix in the chopped cilantro. Serve warm.

Makes 2 servings

Per serving: 374 calories, 15 g fat, 489 mg sodium, 46 g carbs, 9 g fiber, 16 g protein

Chinese Chicken Salad

What you'll need

1   head napa cabbage
⅔   head red cabbage
½   Tbsp sugar
2   cups chopped or shredded cooked chicken (freshly grilled or from a store-bought rotisserie chicken)
⅓   cup Asian Vinaigrette (see below)
1   cup fresh cilantro leaves
1   cup canned mandarin oranges packed in water, drained
¼   cup sliced almonds, toasted
Salt and black pepper, to taste

How to make it

- Slice the cabbages in half lengthwise and remove the cores. Slice the cabbage into thin strips. Toss with the sugar in a large bowl.

- If the chicken is cold, toss with a few tablespoons of vinaigrette and heat in a microwave at 50 percent power. Add to the cabbage, along with the cilantro, mandarins, almonds, and the remaining vinaigrette. Toss to combine. Season with salt and pepper.

Makes 4 servings

Per serving: 392 calories, 21 g fat, 26 g carbs, 4 g fiber, 30 g protein

Asian Vinaigrette

What you'll need

1   Tbsp Dijon mustard
½   Tbsp soy sauce (use a low-sodium variety)
2   Tbsp rice wine vinegar
½   Tbsp toasted sesame oil
¼   cup peanut oil
1   tsp sugar

How to make it

Mix all ingredients together.

Makes 4 servings

Chicken Portobello Wrap

What you'll need

½	medium bell pepper
1	clove garlic, minced
1	Tbsp reduced-fat mayonnaise
1	tsp balsamic vinegar
1	whole-wheat tortilla
2	Tbsp shredded mozzarella
1	small handful mixed greens
1	cup chopped rotisserie chicken or leftover chicken
1	cup Roasted Vegetables

How to make it

- Chop the pepper into ½-inch pieces.

- Mix the garlic, mayonnaise, and vinegar to make the aioli.

- Brush the tortilla with the aioli, then put the cheese down the middle, followed by the greens, chicken, and vegetables. To make a tight wrap, fold the bottom of the tortilla up first, then roll it from the side.

Makes 1 serving with Roasted Vegetables

Per serving: 478 calories, 12 g fat, 418 mg sodium, 42 g carbs, 8 g fiber, 52 g protein

Roasted Vegetables

What you'll need

¾	bunch asparagus (about 8 spears)
3	portobello mushroom caps, sliced ¼" thick
2	onions, cut in ¼"-thick rings
½	Tbsp extra-virgin olive oil

How to make it

- In a baking dish, toss the vegetables with the oil and season with salt and pepper.

- Roast for 15 to 20 minutes, until the vegetables have developed a light brown crust.

Minestrone with Pesto

What you'll need

1   Tbsp olive oil
1   medium onion, chopped
2   cloves garlic, minced
8   oz Yukon gold or red potatoes, cubed
2   medium carrots, peeled and chopped
1   medium zucchini, chopped
8   oz green beans, ends trimmed, halved
Salt and black pepper, to taste
1   14-oz can diced tomatoes
8   cups low-sodium chicken stock
½   tsp dried thyme
½   16-oz can white beans, drained
Pesto, to top
Parmesan, to garnish

How to make it

● Heat the olive oil in a large pot over medium heat. Add the onion and garlic and cook until the onion is translucent, about 3 minutes.

● Stir in the potatoes, carrots, zucchini, and green beans. Season with a bit of salt and cook, stirring, for 3 to 4 minutes to release the vegetables' aromas.

● Add the tomatoes, stock, and thyme and turn the heat down to low. Season with salt and pepper to taste. Simmer for at least 15 minutes, and up to 45.

● Before serving, stir in the white beans and heat through. Serve with a dollop of pesto and bit of grated Parmesan.

Makes 4 servings

Per serving: 248 calories, 6 g fat, 411 mg sodium, 42 g carbs, 9 g fiber, 13 g protein

Lemon Kale Protein Detox

What you'll need

½   lemon, peeled and seeded
½   cup unsweetened almond milk
½   frozen banana
1   cup kale
1   scoop plain plant-based protein powder
3   ice cubes
Water to blend (optional)

How to make it

Place all ingredients in a blender and pulse until blended.

Makes 1 serving

Per serving: 239 calories, 5 g fat, 20 g carbs, 399 mg sodium, 32 g carbs, 9 g fiber, 26 g protein

DINNER RECIPES

Roasted Chicken, Vegetables, and Quinoa

What you'll need

2   skin-on chicken breasts
2   Tbsp olive oil, plus extra
Salt and pepper, to taste
Dried rosemary, to taste
1   medium onion
½   lb red peppers
1 lb carrots
½   lb brussels sprouts
2   cloves garlic
1   package of quinoa

How to make it

- Preheat oven to 400°F.

- Put the chicken breasts on a baking sheet, coating with olive oil, salt, pepper, and dried rosemary, to taste.

- Chop up the vegetables and toss to coat in 2 tablespoons of olive oil and the garlic. Season with salt and pepper. Throw everything on one tray and cook for 25 to 30 minutes, or until chicken reaches an internal temperature of 165°F. Cook the quinoa according to package instructions.

Makes 4 servings

Per serving: 522 calories, 14 g fat (2 g saturated), 263 mg sodium, 76 g carbs, 18 g fiber, 25 g protein

Chicken Salad Sandwich with Curry and Raisins

What you'll need

3   Tbsp golden raisins
3   cups cooked chicken, chopped
2   stalks celery, thinly sliced
½   onion, diced
1   carrot, shredded
½   tsp curry powder
¼   cup olive-oil mayonnaise
Salt and black pepper, to taste
4   large lettuce leaves (romaine, iceberg, or another favorite)
8   slices whole-grain bread or English muffin halves, toasted
2   medium tomatoes, sliced

How to make it

● Cover the raisins with hot water and soak for at least 10 minutes (the warm water will help the raisins plump up); drain and place in a large bowl.

● Add the chicken, celery, onion, carrot, curry powder, and mayonnaise. Mix well and season with salt and pepper.

● Place the lettuce leaves on top of 4 bread slices, then top with the tomatoes, the chicken salad, and the remaining slices of bread.

Makes 4 servings

Per serving: 499 calories, 18 g fat, 708 mg sodium, 49 g carbs, 6 g fiber, 31 g protein

Turkey Bolognese with Spaghetti Squash

What you'll need

1   medium spaghetti squash

1   bulb garlic

3   Tbsp extra-virgin olive oil

1   lb ground turkey

1   cup finely chopped carrots

½   cup finely chopped onion

½   cup finely chopped celery

4   cloves garlic, minced

3   Tbsp tomato paste

½   cup dry red wine

1   8-oz can crushed tomatoes

1   tsp dried oregano, crushed

1   tsp dried basil, crushed

1   tsp fennel seeds, lightly crushed

¾   tsp salt

¾   tsp black pepper

½   cup reduced-sodium chicken broth

How to make it

● Preheat oven to 375°F. Halve the squash lengthwise and scrape out the seeds. Place squash halves, cut side down, in a large baking dish. Prick skin all over with a fork. Cut ½ inch off the top of the head of garlic. Place, cut end up, in the baking dish with the squash. Drizzle with 1 tablespoon of the oil. Bake 35 to 45 minutes, or until squash and garlic are tender.

● While squash is baking, heat 1 tablespoon of the oil in a large pot over medium heat. Add turkey, carrots, onion, celery, and garlic. Cook until turkey is cooked through and vegetables are tender, stirring with a wooden spoon to break up the meat.

- Add tomato paste, cook and stir for 1 minute. Add red wine, tomatoes, oregano, basil, fennel, and ½ teaspoon each of salt and pepper. Add broth and bring to a boil. Reduce heat and simmer, uncovered, for 30 minutes.

- Using a fork, remove and shred the flesh from each squash half, forming spaghetti-like strands. Transfer to a bowl and cover to keep warm. When garlic is cool enough to handle, squeeze the bulb from the bottom to pop out the cloves into a small bowl. Add the remaining 1 tablespoon of oil to the garlic. Mash with a fork. Stir the mashed garlic into the spaghetti squash and season with the remaining salt and pepper.

- Serve with the meat sauce over the spaghetti squash.

Makes 4 servings

Per serving: 370 calories, 12 g fat (3 g saturated), 440 mg sodium, 18 g carbs, 8 g fiber, 22 g protein

Pork Fried Rice

What you'll need

2   4-oz portions of pork

½ cup diced onion

1   Tbsp canola oil

1   cup frozen peas

1   cup frozen carrots

¼ cup frozen corn

1   cup brown rice, cooked

1   Tbsp soy sauce (use a low-sodium variety)

Splash of sesame oil

How to make it

- Cut up the pork into cubes and combine with the diced onion.
- Heat the canola oil in a pan over medium-high heat. Add the pork and onions and sauté for 3 minutes.
- Add the vegetables. Move them to one side of the pan and crack two eggs on the other side, whisking to scramble.
- Add the rice, soy sauce, and a splash of sesame oil and fry together for another minute.

Makes 2 servings

Per serving: 422 calories,15 g fat, 798 mg sodium, 57 g carbs, 7 g fiber, 31 g protein

Asian Slaw

What you'll need

Juice of 1 lime

1   Tbsp olive oil mayonnaise

1   Tbsp sugar

1   tsp Asian-style chili sauce like sriracha

1   tsp sesame oil

8   cups shredded cabbage (preferably a mix of purple and napa cabbage)

1   large carrot, peeled and grated

1   Tbsp sesame seeds

Salt and pepper, to taste

How to make it

In a large salad bowl, mix together the lime juice, mayonnaise, sugar, chili sauce, and sesame oil. Add the cabbage, carrots, and sesame seeds and toss to combine. Season with salt and pepper.

Makes 4–6 servings

Per serving: 103 calories, 4 g fat, 116 mg sodium, 17 g carbs, 5 g fiber, 3 g protein

Creamy Tomato Basil Soup

What you'll need

2   Tbsp olive oil
12   plum tomatoes, halved
1   large sweet onion, coarsely chopped
4   garlic cloves
Salt and pepper, to taste
2   cups low-sodium vegetable stock
1   cup plain Greek yogurt
¼   cup basil, shredded

How to make it

● Preheat an oven to 425°F.

● While oven is heating, combine olive oil, tomatoes, onions, garlic, salt, and pepper in a bowl and toss until the vegetables are fully coated.

● Transfer the mixture to a roasting pan and bake for 25 minutes, or until browned.

● After the veggies are cooked, put them in a soup pot. Add the vegetable stock and bring the mixture to a boil.

● Reduce heat and simmer for about 5 minutes. Next, put the mixture into a blender or food processor and puree along with the yogurt. Add the basil during the last few pulses to combine.

Makes 2 servings

Per serving: 315 calories, 14 g fat, 260 mg sodium, 35 g carbs, 8 g fiber, 17 g protein

Turkey Burger Mediterranean Style

What you'll need

1   lb lean ground turkey
Salt and pepper, to taste
½   tsp dried thyme
½   cup feta or fresh goat cheese
2   cups arugula
4   English muffins, split and lightly toasted (choose whole-grain ones)
½   cup roasted red peppers
¼   cup olives, chopped

How to make it

- Preheat a grill or grill pan.

- Season turkey with a few big pinches of salt and pepper, plus the dried thyme.

- Form the meat into 4 patties, being careful not to overwork the meat (which will cause the proteins to bind, making for a tough burger). Use your thumb to make a small impression in the middle of each patty (as they cook, the middle will swell up; this simple step makes for a more evenly cooked burger.)

- Cook over medium-high heat for 4 to 5 minutes on the first side, until lightly charred. Flip and immediately add the cheese to each patty. Cook for another 4 to 5 minutes, until the burgers feel firm and springy to the touch. Remove from the grill.

- Lay the arugula on the bottom of the English muffin halves. Top with the burger, then crown the burger with peppers, olives, and the other half of the English muffin.

Makes 4 servings

Per serving: 371 calories, 19 g fat, 910 mg sodium, 26 g carbs, 2 g fiber, 21 g protein

Baked Sweet Potato Fries

What you'll need

2   medium sweet potatoes, peeled and cut into wedges
1   Tbsp olive oil
Pinch of cayenne
1   tsp smoked paprika (optional)
Salt and black pepper, to taste

How to make it

- Preheat the oven to 425°F.

- Combine all the ingredients, plus a generous amount of salt and pepper, on a baking sheet and toss to coat evenly.

- Bake until the sweet potatoes have browned on the outside, are crisp to the touch, and are tender inside, about 25 minutes.

Makes 4 servings

Per serving: 95 calories, 4 g fat, 37 mg of sodium, 15 carbs, 2 g fiber, 1 g protein

Sweet and Sour Onions

What you'll need

1 bag (16 oz) frozen pearl onions
¾ cup water
¾ cup white wine or red wine vinegar
¼ cup sugar
Pinch of red pepper flakes
Salt and black pepper, to taste

How to make it

- Combine the onions, water, vinegar, sugar, and pepper flakes in a medium saucepan.

- Place over medium-low heat, cover, and cook for 10 minutes.

- Remove the lid and cook for another 10 minutes, until the liquid has reduced and begins to cling to the onions. The onions should be tender but not falling apart. Season with salt and pepper.

Makes 4 servings

Per serving: 68 calories, 0 g fat, 25 mg sodium, 17 g carbs, 1 g fiber, 0 g protein

Chicken Fajitas

What you'll need

2 Tbsp olive oil
4 boneless skinless chicken breasts, cut into thin strips
Chili powder, ground cumin, and garlic powder, to taste
1–2 packages frozen peppers and onions
Whole grain tortillas
Shredded romaine, lime wedges, and salsa, to taste

How to make it

- Heat 1 tablespoon of the oil in a skillet over medium-high heat. Add chicken, cover the meat in the spices, and cook until it's no longer pink. Remove chicken from skillet and keep warm on a plate.

- In the same skillet, heat the remaining oil over medium-high heat; stir in frozen veggies and cook until vegetables are crisp-tender.

- Spoon chicken and veggies onto the center of each tortilla and serve with lettuce, lime, and salsa.

Makes 4 servings

Per serving: 510 calories, 19 g fat, 426 g sodium, 40 g carbs, 1 g fiber, 48 g protein

Pumpkin Turkey Chili

Recipe by Erin Peisach

What you'll need

2	Tbsp extra-virgin olive oil
2	cups chopped onion
3	garlic cloves, minced (about 3 tsp)
2	cups chopped carrots
1½	cups chopped celery
2	lbs lean ground turkey
1	tsp chili powder
1	tsp dried oregano
2	tsp cumin
2	bay leaves
1	15-oz can white northern beans, rinsed and drained
2	cups broth (low-sodium vegetable or chicken)
1	15-oz can pumpkin puree

Salt and pepper, to taste

How to make it

- In a large stockpot over medium-high heat, add oil. Toss in the onion and garlic and heat for about 5 minutes. Toss in the carrots and celery and heat for an additional 5 minutes.

- Add the ground turkey to the pot and break it up with a wooden spoon. Allow the turkey to brown for about 5 minutes. Add the seasonings, beans, broth, and pumpkin puree and then mix the chili until all of the ingredients are well combined.

- Cover the pot and reduce the heat to medium-low. Allow the chili to simmer for at least 45 minutes.

- Serve warm with additional toppings like sour cream, shredded cheese, cilantro, or diced avocado.

Makes 8 servings

Recipe by Erin Peisach.

Per serving: 242 calories, 5 g fat, 212 mg sodium, 18 g carbs, 3 g fiber, 24 g protein

Fettuccine with Chicken and Roasted Vegetables

What you'll need

3   oz 100 percent whole-wheat fettuccine
½   Tbsp canola oil
1   cup chopped rotisserie chicken
1   cup roasted vegetables*
1½   Tbsp jarred, sun-dried-tomato pesto
Salt and black pepper, to taste
Parmesan cheese
1   cup mixed greens, drizzled with olive oil and balsamic vinegar

How to make it

● Cook the fettuccine according to the package directions. Drain.

● Mix the chicken, vegetables, and pesto with the pasta. Season with salt and pepper.

● Grate some Parmesan and sprinkle on top. Serve with the greens.

Makes 1 serving

Per serving: 709 calories, 21 g fat, 749 mg sodium, 94 g carbs, 20 g fiber, 41 g protein

San Antonio Rice Bowl

What you'll need

Rice, beans, and fajita mix saved from the Shrimp Fajitas recipe
½   avocado, peeled and thinly sliced
Salsa (optional)

How to make it

Heat the leftovers in a plastic container or a microwaveable bowl for 60 seconds. Top with the avocado and salsa to taste, if desired.

Makes 1 serving

Per serving: 319 calories, 19 g fat, 467 mg sodium, 23 g carbs, 27 g fiber, 32 g protein

Shrimp Fajitas

What you'll need

¼   cup instant brown rice
½   can black beans, drained and heated
½   Tbsp canola or other cooking oil
1   onion, sliced
1   cup chopped bell pepper
2   garlic cloves, chopped
8   oz frozen shrimp, defrosted
Cayenne pepper, crushed red pepper, or Tabasco, to taste
½   tsp cumin
Salt and black pepper, to taste
½   avocado, pitted, peeled, and thinly sliced
1   whole-wheat tortilla, warmed

How to make it

- Cook the rice according to the package directions, then add the beans.

- Heat the oil in a large skillet or wok over high heat. Add the onion, the bell pepper, and garlic; cook for 5 to 7 minutes, until the vegetables begin to brown.

- Mix in the shrimp and spices; cook for another 3 minutes, until the shrimp are pink and firm.

- Serve half of the shrimp fajita mix with a small scoop of the rice and beans, the avocado slices, and the tortilla.

- Reserve the rest of the rice and beans in a microwavable bowl or plastic container along with the leftover fajita mix and use them for tomorrow's lunch. Wrap the leftover avocado well and refrigerate to minimize browning.

Makes 1 serving

Per serving: 438 calories, 18 g fat, 609 mg sodium, 53 g carbs, 22 g fiber, 37 g protein

Bluefish with Potatoes

What you'll need

1   lb Yukon Gold potatoes
1   Tbsp kosher salt
1   cup plain Greek yogurt
1   tsp fresh lemon juice
1   tsp white wine vinegar
¾   tsp ground black pepper
4   cloves garlic, peeled, crushed
5   Tbsp extra-virgin olive oil, divided
4   6-oz skin-on bluefish (or mackerel) fillets
2   Tbsp fresh oregano leaves
1   tsp finely grated lemon zest
Sea salt and black pepper, to taste

How to make it

- Place potatoes in a large pot and cover with water. Season with kosher salt. Bring to a boil, reduce heat, and simmer for 10 to 12 minutes. Drain; let cool.

- Preheat a broiler. Whisk yogurt, lemon juice, and vinegar in a bowl. Season with kosher salt and pepper.

- Place potatoes in a rimmed baking sheet that can be used in a broiler. Smash the potatoes flat with the bottom of a heavy measuring cup. Add garlic and 4 tablespoons of the oil, and toss the potatoes to coat. Season with kosher salt and black pepper. Broil the potatoes for 12 minutes, or until golden brown.

- Rub skin side of fish with remaining oil; season with kosher salt and black pepper. Place, skin side up, on top of smashed potatoes and broil until fish is cooked and skin is crispy, about 10 minutes.

- Remove from oven, top with oregano and lemon zest. Spoon yogurt sauce into each plate and place potatoes and fish on the sauce. Sprinkle with sea salt.

Makes 4 servings

Per serving: 655 calories, 40 g fat, 310 mg sodium, 20 g carbs, 3 g fiber, 39 g protein

Cedar Plank Salmon

What you'll need

2   Tbsp grainy mustard
2   Tbsp light brown sugar
½   Tbsp fresh thyme leaves (or 1 tsp dried thyme)
1   large salmon fillet
1   large cedar plank, soaked in water for 30 minutes
Salt and pepper, to taste

How to make it

● Preheat a grill over medium-low heat.

● Combine the mustard, brown sugar, and thyme in a bowl.

● Place the salmon, skin side down, on top of the cedar plank, season with salt and pepper, and spread the mustard mixture on the top.

● Place the plank directly on the grill grate and close the lid. Grill for about 20 minutes, until the center of the fillet flakes with gentle pressure from the finger and an instant-read thermometer inserted into the thickest part of the salmon registers 135°F.

Makes 4 servings

Per serving: 301 calories, 13 g fat, 312 mg sodium, 6 g carbs, 0 g fiber, 29 g protein

Roasted Parmesan Asparagus

What you'll need

1   bunch asparagus, about 1½ lbs
1   Tbsp olive oil
2   Tbsp grated Parmesan
Salt and black pepper, to taste
Juice of 1 lemon

How to make it

● Preheat the oven to 400°F.

● Hold an asparagus spear at both ends and bend the bottom until the tough, woody section snaps (it will naturally snap off where the tough part of the vegetable ends and the tender part begins.) Using that spear as a guide, use a knife to remove the bottoms of the rest of the bunch.

● Place the asparagus in a baking dish. Drizzle with the olive oil, sprinkle with the Parmesan, and season with salt and pepper; toss to coat. Roast until just tender, 10 to 12 minutes. Sprinkle the lemon juice over the asparagus.

Makes 4 servings

Per serving: 80 calories, 4 g fat, 9 g carbs, tk g fiber, 5 g protein

Baked Halibut

What you'll need

2   5-oz fillets of halibut
1   jar marinated artichoke hearts
1   cup cherry tomatoes
2   Tbsp kalamata olives
½   medium fennel bulb
1   lemon, sliced into eighths
½   Tbsp olive oil
¼   cup dry white wine
Salt and pepper, to taste

How to make it

- Preheat the oven to 400°F.

- Take 2 large sheets of parchment paper or foil, place a fillet in the center of each, and top equally with the artichokes, tomatoes, olives, fennel, and lemon slices. Drizzle with the olive oil and wine; season with salt and pepper. Fold the paper or foil over the fish and seal by tightly rolling up the edges, creating a secure pouch. It's important that the packets are fully sealed so that the steam created inside can't escape.

- Place the pouches on a baking sheet in the center of the oven and bake for 20 to 25 minutes, depending on how thick the fish is. Serve with the remaining lemon wedges.

Makes 2 servings

Per serving: 296 calories, 10 g fat, 444 mg sodium, 11 g carbs, 5 g fiber, 33 g protein

SNACK RECIPES

Chocolate-Covered Strawberries

What you'll need

6 oz semisweet chocolate (chips or bar)
20 strawberries, stems left on, rinsed, and blotted dry
20 toothpicks

How to make it

- Place the chocolate chips in a microwave-safe bowl and microwave until melted. Stir every 30 seconds. Set aside to cool slightly.

- Line a plate or rimmed baking sheet with parchment paper.

- Insert a toothpick into the stem of each strawberry. Dip the strawberries in the melted chocolate, turning to coat.

- Place the dipped strawberries on the lined plate and refrigerate until the chocolate hardens, about 20 minutes. Serve chilled.

Makes 20 servings

Per serving: 138 calories, 3 g fat, 4 mg sodium, 29 g carbs, 7 g fiber, 2 g protein

Awesome Guacamole

What you'll need

¼   cup cilantro
2   cloves garlic, minced
Salt, to taste
2   ripe avocados, pitted and peeled
¼   cup minced onion
2   Tbsp minced jalapeño pepper
Juice of 1 lemon

How to make it

- Combine the cilantro and garlic on a cutting board and use the back of a chef's knife to work them into a fine paste; a pinch of coarse salt helps this process.

- Transfer the paste to a bowl and add the avocado. Use a fork to smash the avocado into a mostly smooth—but still slightly chunky—puree. Stir in the onion, jalapeño, lemon juice, and a bit more salt.

Makes 4 servings

Per serving: 211 calories, 12 g fat, 117 mg sodium, 28 g carbs, 13 g fiber, 4 g protein

Hummus with Celery and Cucumbers

What you'll need

1   15-oz can chickpeas
1   clove garlic
2   tsp ground cumin
Juice of 1 lemon
¾   tsp salt
2   Tbsp tahini
¼   cup olive oil
Sprinkle of paprika
½   cup celery and cucumber sticks

How to make it

● Drain and rinse the chickpeas and throw them into a blender. Add the garlic, cumin, lemon juice, salt, and tahini. Blend.

● While blending, slowly drizzle in ¼ cup of olive oil until smooth and creamy. Top with a sprinkle of paprika before serving. Use as a dip with celery and cucumber sticks.

Makes 6 servings

Per serving: 363 calories, 17 g fat (2.3 g saturated fat), 315 mg sodium, 42 g carbs, 11 g fiber, 13 g protein

Low-FODMAP Snack Balls

Recipe by Erin Peisach

These snacks are formulated to fit with Low-FODMAP diets, which are special diets designed to minimize digestive issues. FODMAP stands for fermentable oligo, di, monosaccharides, and polyols. All you have to remember is that these types of carbs can trigger bloating and gas. These snacks minimize those symptoms and, so, they fit perfectly into our plan.

What you'll need

¼   cup dry old fashioned oats
¼   cup pecan or walnut halves
2   Tbsp chia seeds
2   Tbsp hemp seeds
¼   cup unsweetened coconut flakes
1   Tbsp coconut oil, melted
2   Tbsp maple syrup
½   tsp vanilla extract
¼   cup almond meal

How to make it

● Add the oats and the pecans/walnuts into a food processor or blender and pulse until well combined.

● Add the rest of the ingredients into the food processor or blender and pulse until well combined.

● Place the batter into a mixing bowl. Begin rolling the batter into ping pong–size balls and place in a separate container. Store the snack balls in a closed container in the refrigerator.

Makes 6 balls
Per serving: (2 balls): 175 calories, 13 g fat, 11 g carbs, 3 g fiber, 4.5 g protein

How to Make Low-Sodium Salad Dressings

A quick salad is one of the best delivery vessels for your daily vegetables (and sometimes fruits, too.) To make salads extra special, try these delicious healthy dressings.

Citrus Tahini

2   Tbsp tahini
1   Tbsp apple cider vinegar
2   Tbsp fresh lemon juice
2   Tbsp fresh orange juice
2   Tbsp honey
1   tsp dijon mustard
Salt and pepper, to taste

Makes 10 servings

Per serving: 33 calories, 2 g fat, 0 g saturated fat, 42 mg sodium, 5 g carbs, 0 g fiber, 1 g protein

Raspberry Vinaigrette

¼   cup raspberries
¼   cup white wine vinegar
¼   cup apple cider vinegar
½   cup olive oil
1   Tbsp honey

Makes 10 servings

Per serving: 103 calories, 11 g fat, 1 g saturated fat, 4 mg sodium, 3 g carbs, 0 g fiber, 0 g protein

Avo Goddess

½   medium avocado
½   cup Greek yogurt
½   cup water
3   Tbsp fresh lime juice
1   cup fresh cilantro
1   clove garlic
1   tsp onion powder
Pinch of salt

Makes 6 servings

Per serving: 20 calories, 1 g fat, 0 g saturated fat, 6 mg sodium, 3 g carbs, 1 g fiber, 1 g protein

Sweet Pomegranate Vinaigrette

1   cup pomegranate juice
¼   cup honey
1   Tbsp Dijon mustard
⅓   cup olive oil
½   cup pomegranate seeds

Makes 10 servings

Per serving: 112 calories, 7 g fat, 1 g saturated fat, 29 mg sodium, 12 g carbs, 0.3 g fiber, 0 g protein

Asian Peanut Dressing

¼   cup unsalted peanut butter
1   Tbsp soy sauce
2   Tbsp honey
1   Tbsp lime
½   tsp chili garlic sauce
Hot water for consistency

Makes 10 servings

Per serving: 60 calories, 3 g fat, 1 g saturated fat, 66 mg sodium, 6 g carbs, 1 g fiber, 2 g protein

11

What's Next

Here's how to keep pace on your lifelong journey from Day 8 on.

E HOPE you've enjoyed the last 7 days on the Healthy Heart Diet program, and we encourage you to keep the momentum going. Day 8 shouldn't be different than yesterday, and the journey to a healthier heart doesn't stop at the back cover of this book. Keep eating right, moving more, prioritizing sleep, and doing your best to protect your heart.

In the days and weeks to come, you will encounter more opportunities to make heart-smart choices that might not have come up in Days 1 through Day 7. Here are some other suggestions to support a healthier heart:

Get recommended vaccines

Flu vaccinations are important, and not just for elderly folks and children. A recent study published in *the New England Journal of Medicine* suggests that your chances of suffering a heart attack increase six-fold during the first seven days after being diagnosed with the flu. In other words, a yearly flu shot is a smart investment in bulletproofing your heart. Another vaccine to consider is the shingles shot. Shingles, which originates from the chicken pox virus, is an itchy, scabby, painful ailment that can be more than a nuisance. In a study from South Korea, people who had shingles were 41 percent more likely to have a cardiovascular event, with 59 percent having an increased risk for heart attack and 35 percent, for stroke.

Visit your dentist twice yearly

Poor dental hygiene is more than a cosmetic problem. People who go to the dentist and have their teeth cleaned have a lower risk of heart attack and stroke than people who never do, according to research from Taiwan. One explanation is that people who neglect their teeth are more likely to develop gum disease, a condition that encourages your immune cells to secrete inflammatory molecules that might harm your heart. If you haven't seen your dentist in a while, make an appointment, and in the meantime, invest in a toothbrush with a timer, or at least one you like using. People who brush less than twice a day or for less than two minutes per session have an increased risk of low flow-mediated dilation, a measure of how well blood vessels constrict and expand, according to new research in the *International Journal of Cardiology*. And don't forget to floss!

Go easy on pain relievers

We all take the occasional pain reliever for a pounding headache or an achy back, but ibuprofen and other non-steroidal anti-inflammatory drugs (NSAIDs) are not made to be popped willy-nilly. In a recent study, researchers in Canada found that people taking NSAIDs every day were 20 to 50 percent more likely to suffer a heart attack down the road than those who didn't. These drugs inhibit an enzyme called cyclooxygenase 2, which has some heart-protecting benefits. People on the higher end of the risk spectrum took about 1,200 milligrams of ibuprofen—or about roughly six tablets of basic Advil or Motrin—every day or about 750 milligrams of Naproxen, the active ingredient in Aleve. Tylenol, which is not an NSAID, might be safer for your heart. But if you have so much pain that you consider popping six Advils a day every day for weeks at a time, talk to a doctor about alternative strategies. Depending on the cause of your pain, you might benefit from another intervention, such as physical therapy.

4

Number of extra years lived on average by people who had zero cardiovascular risk factors at age 44

Source: *Circulation*

Recognize depression

Our minds and hearts work in tandem, and a problem with one could spell trouble for the other. Depression, anxiety, and other mental health problems have been linked to cardiovascular disease, and scientists have multiple theories about why this might be true. For example, depression might increase inflammation in your body and harm your heart. Anxiety might turn up your sympathetic nervous system in a way that can make your blood vessels less flexible and less resilient over time, making them more prone to clots and ruptures. The good news is that many of the same strategies that can calm your mind, such as meditation, might help your heart at the same time.

Test your ticker

These 10 tests can give your doctor and you a wealth of information about your cardiovascular health.

1. Blood pressure test. As your blood moves through your body, it presses against the walls of your blood vessels. Too much pressure can wear down your system, while too little can signal a different serious problem. What's scary is 16 percent of American adults with high blood pressure don't know they have it, according to the American Heart Association. Find out your BP the next time you visit the doctor's office; often a nurse or medical assistant will take it at the beginning of the visit. In the meantime, you can check it at a local pharmacy. Many now have automated machines that will tell you your pressure for free. If it's in a range that signals you it needs watching, you can buy an electronic device to monitor yourself at home. Your numbers should be under 130/80. If they are high, your doctor might put you on a low-sodium diet and prescribe medications to bring the pressure down.

2. Cholesterol panel Cholesterol, little fats floating in your bloodstream, can go rogue, attach to the walls of your vessels, and build up. When your arteries are hardened and narrowed by these cholesterol plaques, your risk of a heart attack spikes. Your doctor will probably check your cholesterol numbers about every five years and maybe more often if you have certain risk factors such as heart disease, diabetes, or kidney problems. Your total cholesterol should be less than 200 mg/dL, and your LDL, commonly considered the "bad" cholesterol, should be less than 100 mg/dL. Your HDL, or the "good" cholesterol, should be 60 mg/dL or higher. Triglycerides, another type of fat in your bloodstream, will be measured at the same time, and they should come in at less than 150 mg/dL. If your numbers are high, your doctor might prescribe cholesterol-lowering statins.

3. Lipoprotein[a] Also known as "Lp Little a," this is a more advanced test of blood fats that looks to measure a protein attached to LDL particles that encourages LDL to infiltrate coronary artery walls. This protein is inherited. LPa can help predict cardiovascular risk above and beyond cholesterol, especially in people at intermediate risk, research suggest.

4. Blood sugar tests A blood glucose test can tell you a lot about your heart. Diabetes, a condition marked by high blood sugar and difficulty producing the metabolic hormone insulin, can damage your cardiovascular system and raise your risk of heart disease or a stroke. Research published in the journal *The Lancet* suggests that people with type 2 diabetes have an increased risk of various heart problems, from peripheral artery disease to strokes to angina to heart failure to heart attacks.

Diabetes is one of the most commonly diagnosed

ailments in the world, with 30.3 million individuals—that's 9.4 percent of the U.S. population—dealing with the disease in the United States alone. Scarier yet is that 7.2 million diabetics in the United States don't even realize they have it. While discovering you have diabetes can be a terrifying prospect, the sooner you're treated, the more manageable your condition will be. In fact, a review of research published in the American Diabetes Association journal *Diabetes Care* reveals that early treatment with insulin can help patients with type 2 diabetes manage their blood sugar better and gain less weight than those who start treatment later.

Ask your doctor to check your blood glucose levels. A normal result is 100 mg/dL after eight hours of fasting. If your blood sugar measures 100 to 125 mg/dL, you are in the prediabetic range. Weight loss can sometimes bring you into the safe zone. If your blood sugar is 126 mg/dL or higher, you fall into the diabetes zone and your doctor may recommend medication to manage your sugar.

Another useful diabetes test is the hemoglobin A1C blood test, HbA1C for short. It measures your average blood sugar over two to three months. This can give you more insight than a single fasting blood sugar reading. Ask for it if you are 45 or older—or you are younger but overweight and have one or more diabetes or heart disease risk factors.

5. Echocardiogram This ultrasound of the heart helps a doctor view your ticker's structure, detect heart-valve problems, and measure pumping function. A key measure of heart health is ejection fraction, the percentage of blood expelled by the left ventricle during each heartbeat. A left ventricle that's functioning well pumps about 60 percent with each beat. This test might be appropriate if you have a heart valve problem, murmur, or history of heart attack. Lower percentages of blood pumped by the left ventricle may indicate increased risk of congestive heart failure.

6. C-reactive protein This protein, also called CRP, can be an early indicator of inflammation in your body. High levels can be a warning sign that your heart is at risk. Your doctor can check this by ordering a blood test. A good result is 3 milligrams per deciliter or lower.

7. Homocysteine A blood test measures levels of this abrasive amino acid, which irritates the lining of arteries, opening them up to infiltration by LDL and leading to plaque and blood clotting. One study showed that high homocysteine levels lead to an increase in stroke risk comparable to the risk of a pack-a-day smoker. The test can signal a doctor to prescribe folate, vitamin B6, and vitamin B12 supplements, which can help to reduce homocysteine.

8. CT scan for calcium score The CT (computerized tomography) scan is a series of x-ray views taken from different angles to create a cross-sectional view of your heart. The scanner can detect calcified plaque in your coronary arteries—a precursor to heart attacks.

9. Endothelial function test A noninvasive test, such as the EndoPAT, analyzes the health of the thin lining of your blood vessels (called the endothelium) and the ability of your blood vessels to dilate. Endothelial dysfunction may be the first observable manifestation of vascular disease.

Stay in the know

To keep up with the latest updates in heart health research and advice through these trusted resources.

The American Heart Association
(heart.org)

Here, you'll find healthy living tips and much more, including CPR training information that could help you save not only your own life, but also someone else's.

On Twitter: @American_Heart
On Facebook: facebook.com/AmericanHeart
On Instagram: american_heart

National Heart, Lung, and Blood Institute
(https://www.nhlbi.nih.gov/).

This unit of the National Institutes of Health aims to understand human biology, reduce disease, develop workforce resources, and advance research. Go here to learn about the latest research on chronic diseases.

On Twitter: @nih_nhlbi
On Facebook: facebook.com/NHLBI

Harvard Health Publishing
(health.harvard.edu/topics/heart-health).

A team from America's oldest higher education institution offers information on heart conditions, symptoms, treatments, and more.

On Twitter: @HarvardHealth
On Facebook: facebook.com/HarvardHealthPublications

Special Report:
What women must know
about heart attacks

When most people think of a heart attack, they envision a man clutching his chest and keeling over.

"We call that the 'Hollywood Heart Attack,'" says Leslie Davis, PhD, RN, an associate professor of nursing at the University of North Carolina–Greensboro. "That's what women expect."

Reality paints a different picture. While chest pain is the most common heart attack symptom, about a third of female heart attack victims don't get chest pain, Davis says. Compared to men, women are more likely to experience shoulder pain, throat pain, back pain, and nausea during heart attacks.

"You're lucky if a heart attack is one of those Hollywood Heart Attacks or gets your attention so you sit up straight in bed," she says. "Those people, men or women, are very likely to call the ambulance or get to the hospital quickly."

Heart attack symptoms can be vague, and they might come and go or evolve, says Davis. Her research suggests that women with these vague types of symptoms waste valuable time before seeking medical attention. Almost half of women take a wait-and-see approach instead of seeking medical attention right away for a heart attack, says Davis. Many men do this too, but on average, women wait an extra half hour.

Heart attacks typically occur over a span of 8 to 12 hours, but every minute of delay in seeking care increases your chances of having complications, including an increased chance of dying.

"If something [feels] different and it just won't go away, then you need to get it checked out, and you need to get it checked out then," says Davis. That's especially true if you have a history of diabetes, high blood pressure, high cholesterol, or if you smoke or are age 55 or older.

If you suspect a heart attack, don't drive yourself to the ER; call an ambulance. The emergency medical technicians can start administering treatments and tests right away so that when you arrive at the hospital, the cardiovascular care team is ready for you.

One more thing: The Easiest and Most Fun Way to Protect Your Heart

Have a party. Hang out with friends. Hug your spouse. Go dancing. Go to church or synagogue. Volunteer. Be social.

All of those things make up the easiest, cheapest and most enjoyable ways to make your heart stronger. A body of research suggests that people who have support from friends and their communities have healthier hearts than loners do. For example, Harvard researchers recently found that the most socially integrated women were 45 percent less likely to develop fatal coronary heart disease than women who were the least socially integrated. Social integration came from a combination of relationships—with a romantic partner, close friends, a religious community, or other community or volunteer groups. These buddies may cheer you on and help you live a healthy lifestyle. Plus, emerging research suggests that social support might help you fend off heart-damaging inflammation.

In other words, bringing a smile to a friend's face could warm your heart and make your heart healthier at the same time. When you think about it, you have oodles of control over your health destiny as far as your heart is concerned. Take the steps now to enjoy a healthier, happier, more active life. For life!

Appendix A

The 30 Worst Foods for Your Heart

LOOK, WE KNOW and you know that you aren't going to eat cardiologist-approved foods every time you lift a fork. That's OK, as long as you focus on heart-healthy foods most mealtimes and do your best to avoid those salty, sugary, saturated fatty foods that are among the worst for your heart health. To help you clean up your diet, we've compiled a handy list of worsts, and, yes, it includes *wurst* (sausage). Consider the following a cheat sheet of really bad-for-you foods you'll want to boot out of your diet ASAP. Why?

BECAUSE THEY'RE HIGH IN SALT

1. Canned Vegetables

The preservatives and sauces that keep the vitamin-filled veggies company inside the container are packed with sodium. Look for "no salt added" or "low sodium" options and be sure to rinse your veggies thoroughly before digging in. Can't find an unsalted option? Consider switching to frozen vegetables; there are plenty of unsalted selections.

2. Restaurant Soup

Get this: P.F. Chang's Hot & Sour Soup Bowl, packs an artery-shivering 3,800 milligrams of sodium. That's more than four days' worth or the equivalent of about 21 individual bags of Cool Ranch Doritos. Many restaurant soups are similarly salty. Our advice: Make soup at home where you can control the sodium.

3. Cold Cuts

According to a *Journal of the Academy of Nutrition and Dietetics* study, nearly half of Americans consume a sandwich every day—one of the top sources of salt in the American diet. Coincidental? No way. Cold cuts and cheese contribute about 250 milligrams of sodium per slice.

4. Tomato Sauce

A half-cup of Hunt's Tomato sauce packs 830 milligrams of sodium—which is more than you'd find in 97 Cheez-It crackers! To reduce the sodium hit, look for jars of tomato sauce with fewer than 350 milligrams per half-cup serving.

5. Frozen Meals

Frozen dinners may be quick and easy options when you're time-strapped, but they're also loaded with sodium. Two prime examples: Lean Cuisine's French Bread Pepperoni Pizza and Special K's Sausage, Egg & Cheese Flatbread Breakfast Sandwich each pack 700 milligrams—or just under half a day's worth. When you're in the freezer aisle, look for meals with less than 500 milligrams per serving.

6. Vegetable Juice

Prefer to sip your greens rather than chew 'em? Stick with the freshly made varieties from a local juice shop (or your kitchen). The bottled versions are filled to the brim with salt. For example, just 8-ounces of V8 Vegetable Juice Essential Antioxidants has 480 milligrams of sodium.

7 & 8. Capers & Ketchup

Condiments are salty. Those capers on top of your Chicken Piccata carry over 200 milligrams of salt per *tablespoon*. And ketchup has 167 milligrams in the same serving size.

9. Cottage Cheese

A one-cup serving can carry almost 700 milligrams of the mineral—more than a third of what you're supposed to have in an entire day. Be wary of how much you eat and consider a switch to a no-salt-added variety, or eat Greek yogurt instead.

10. Beef Jerky

Sure, it's packed with protein, but jerky is also notoriously high in salt. A 1-ounce serving can contain 700 milligrams of salt, more than four times what you'd find in chips.

BECAUSE THEY CAN CLOG YOUR ARTERIES

11. Coffee Creamer

Traditional coffee creamers are prime sources of trans-fats, often hiding under the guise of hydrogenated oil.

12. Baked Pies

Baked desserts are one of the most potent sources of trans-fat in the American diet. One 14-year study of 80,000 women found a positive correlation between heart disease and the consumption of foods containing trans fatty acids.

13. Ice Cream

A healthy adult should consume no more than 300 milligrams of cholesterol a day. A cup of certain Ben and Jerry's flavors contain more than a third of the day's intake (130 grams!)—and so do plenty of other creamy, cool treats.

14. Fried Chicken

A one 4-ounce serving of fried chicken with the skin on it has as much cholesterol as 11 strips of bacon.

15. Margarine

Butter alternatives like margarine are often made with partially hydrogenated oils, one of the most common sources of trans-fats. Skip this high-cholesterol food and stick with heart-healthy olive oil or grass-fed butter .

16. Biscuits

Packaged biscuits—those fluffy pillows that make fried chicken dinners extra delicious—are full of trans fats.

BECAUSE THEY RAISE YOUR BLOOD SUGAR

17. White Rice

While whole grains can reduce your risk of dying of heart disease by nearly 20 percent, nutrient-stripped refined grains have the opposite effect on your health. In one study of more than 350,00 people, those who ate the most white rice were at greatest risk for type 2 diabetes.

18. Blended Coffees

Warning: Blended coffees laced with syrup, sugar, whipped cream, and other toppings can have as many calories and fat grams as a milkshake.

19. Chinese Take-Out

Thanks to their sugary sauces and deep-fried breading, Chinese restaurant favorites like sesame chicken and sweet and sour pork are packed with calories, fat, and sodium.

20. Cinnamon Rolls

All pastries are sugar and carb landmines, but cinnamon rolls may be the very worst of the lot: A Classic Roll from Cinnabon has 880 calories, 127 grams of carbs and 58 grams of sugar—which is about what you'd find in 10 Chips Ahoy! Chewy cookies.

21 & 22. Bacon & Sausage

Many of these meats contain nitrates, a preservative that interferes with the body's natural ability to process sugar, which increases the risk for diabetes. If that wasn't bad enough, most processed meats are also loaded with sodium.

BECAUSE THEY CAUSE WEIGHT GAIN

23. Bouillon Cubes

When made with a homemade stock or low-sodium broth, soup is a healthy, soothing meal. Make the stuff with a bouillon cube, however, and you've got yourself an entirely different bowl of nutrition—one that's overflowing with monosodium glutamate. MSG is a flavoring agent that increases appetite and tells the body to pump out insulin, the fat-storage hormone.

24. Potato Chips

According to Harvard researchers, chips are one of the worst foods for your belly. Not only are they full of saturated fat, they're also crusted with salt—yet another nutrient linked to cardiovascular disease when eaten in excess. In the Harvard study, daily chip consumption alone was responsible for adding nearly two pounds of flab to study participants' frame every four years.

25. Diet Soda

Recent studies have found an association between sipping diet soda and wider waist circumference. It may seem counter-intuitive since your go-to Diet Cherry Pepsi has zero calories, but researchers think diet soda drinkers may overestimate how many calories they're "saving," and then overeat.

26. Cheese

Cheese is the single biggest contributor of saturated fat to the American diet. And unlike other fats, the saturated variety is the most likely to be stored in the stomach and wreak havoc on your cardiovascular well being. Enjoy cheese and its nutritional benefits, but minimize consumption.

27. Pizza

Pizza is the second biggest contributor of saturated fat to the American diet, and most slices serve up half a day's worth of the artery clogger. To keep your health and waistline in check, stick to one slice and pair it with a house salad.

28. French Fries

Consider French fries a triple threat to your heart health. Not only are they filled with simple sources of carbs that can spike your blood sugar, but they're also filled with fat and salt, too. A 20-year Harvard study found that people who regularly ate fries gained more than three pounds every four years. And over the course of the study, the French fry eaters gained 15 pounds of belly flab from fries alone.

29. Steak

Ribeye, T-bone, and New York Strip are three of the fattiest. Stick to grass-fed top sirloin or London broil to keep your heart in top condition.

30. Fruit Juice

It's natural! It's packed with Vitamin C! It comes from Florida! What could be wrong? Well, while 100-percent fruit juice is a better pick than sugary drinks like Sunny D, even the all-natural stuff still packs up to 36 grams of sugar per cup. What's more, most of the sweetness in juice comes from fructose, a type of sugar associated with the development of belly fat.

Appendix B

The Healthy Heart Diet Restaurant Guide

MERICANS LOVE RESTAURANTS. On average, we eat outside the home 18 times a month. That's not a great statistic for your heart health. As you've learned from this book, restaurant fare is loaded with calories, packs megadoses of sodium, and is heavy on saturated fats. We encourage you to cook more of your meals at home so you can be in control of what fuels your body. But we are realistic, too. We know that you will probably never shun restaurants completely. That's OK. You can still protect your heart and health by making smarter choices when you do go out to eat. Check the nutrition info on the menu before ordering and use this list below to guide you to healthier fare.

APPLEBEE'S

EAT THIS!

8-ounce Select Sirloin with Fire-grilled Veggies

Per serving: 730 calories, 24 g fat (9 g saturated), 1,420 mg sodium, 10 g carbs, 6 g sugars, 4 g fiber, 35 g protein

NOT THAT!

Salsa Verde Beef Nachos

Per serving: 1,760 calories, 118 g fat (50 g saturated fat, 5 g trans fat), 6,040 mg sodium, 106 g carbs, 14 g sugars, 8 g fiber, 71 g protein

BOB EVANS

EAT THIS!

Whole-Egg Veggie Omelet with Spinach and Onions

Per serving: 440 calories, 23 g fat (7 g saturated fat), 430 mg sodium, 34 g carbs, 15 g sugars, 4 g fiber, 26 g protein

NOT THAT!

Country Fried Steak and 2 Eggs with Grits, Country Gravy, and 2 Biscuits

Per serving: 1,500 calories, 102 g fat (37 g saturated fat, 2.5 g trans fat), 2,880 mg sodium, 105 g carbs, 4 g sugars, 6 g fiber, 42 g protein

BONEFISH GRILL

EAT THIS!

Cod Piccata

Per serving: 560 calories, 42 g fat (21 g saturated fat, 1.5 g trans fat), 430 mg sodium, 10 g carbs, 2 g sugars, 2 g fiber, 37 g protein

NOT THAT!

Ahi Tuna Poke

Per serving: 540 calories, 30 g fat (3 g saturated fat), 6,700 mg sodium, 43 g carbs, 11 g sugars, 5 g fiber, 26 g protein

BUFFALO WILD WINGS

EAT THIS!

Traditional Wings with Chipotle BBQ Dry Rub

Per serving: 655 calories, 36 g fat (12 g saturated fat, 1 g trans fat), 430 mg sodium, 1 g carbs, 80 g protein

NOT THAT!

Large Spicy Garlic Boneless Wings

Per serving: 1,630 calories, 89 g fat (31 g saturated fat), 7,620 mg sodium, 130 g carbs, 2 g sugars, 12 g fiber, 77 g protein

BURGER KING

EAT THIS!

Whopper Jr.

Per serving: 310 calories, 18 g fat (5 g saturated fat, 0.5 g trans fat), 390 mg sodium, 27 g carbs, 7 g sugar, 1 g fiber, 13 g protein

NOT THAT!

Rodeo King Sandwich

Per serving: 1,250 calories, 82 g fat (31 g saturated fat, 3.5 g trans fat), 2,270 mg sodium, 69 g carbs, 14 g sugars, 3 g fiber, 60 g protein

CALIFORNIA PIZZA KITCHEN

EAT THIS!

Banh Mi Bowl

Per serving: 540 calories, 33 g fat (4.5 g saturated fat, 0 g trans fat), 770 mg sodium, 40 g carbs, 10 g sugars, 9 g fiber, 28 g protein

NOT THAT!

Jamaican Jerk Chicken Thin Crust Pizza, 1 pie

Per serving: 1,320 calories, 42 g fat (18 g saturated fat), 3,960 mg sodium, 162 g carbs, 36 g sugars, 6 g fiber, 72 g protein

CARRABBA'S ITALIAN GRILL

EAT THIS!

Tuscan Strawberry Salad with Chicken

Per serving: 516 calories, 32 g fat (7 g saturated fat), 781 mg sodium, 24 g carbs, 13 g sugars, 8 g fiber, 35 g protein

NOT THAT!

Fettuccine Weesie

Per serving: 1,510 calories, 95 g fat (62 g saturated fat, 2 g trans fat), 3,430 mg sodium, 98 g carbs, 6 g sugars, 8 g fiber, 58 g protein

CHILI'S BAR & GRILL

EAT THIS!

Original BBQ Ribs, Half Rack

Per serving: 710 calories, 53 g fat (20 g saturated fat), 960 mg sodium, 10 g carbs, 9 g sugars, 49 g protein

NOT THAT!

Crispy Fiery Pepper Crispers

Per serving: 1,750 calories, 91 g fat (15 g saturated fat), 5,790 mg sodium, 179 g carbs, 55 g sugars, 13 g fiber, 58 g protein

DENNY'S

EAT THIS!

Fit Slam Egg White Scramble with Spinach and Grape Tomatoes, Turkey Bacon, English Muffin, and Fruit

Per serving: 390 calories, 10 g fat (2 g saturated fat), 890 mg sodium, 54 g carbs, 17 g sugars, 6 g fiber, 24 g protein

NOT THAT!

The Grand Slamwich with Hash Browns

Per serving: 1,290 calories, 82 g fat (27 g saturated fat, 1 g trans fat), 3,310 mg sodium, 87 g carbs, 10 g sugars, 3 g fiber, 51 g protein

HOOTERS

EAT THIS!
12 Piece Buffalo Shrimp

Per serving: 410 calories, 22 g fat (4 g saturated fat), 820 mg sodium, 25 g carbs, 4 g sugars, 4 g fiber, 29 g protein

NOT THAT!
DD Burger

Per serving: 1,690 calories, 94 g fat (37 g saturated fat, 4.5 g trans fat), 4,960 mg sodium, 111 g carbs, 12 g sugars, 10 g fiber, 93 g protein

IHOP

EAT THIS!
Banana Crepe with Nutella

Per serving: 490 calories, 14 g fat (18 g saturated fat), 450 mg sodium, 61 g carbs, 34 g sugars, 3 g fiber, 11 g protein

NOT THAT!
Buttermilk Biscuits and Gravy with Sausage Gravy

Per serving: 1,370 calories, 93 g fat (138 g saturated fat), 3,480 mg sodium, 196 g carbs, 5 g sugars, 4 g fiber, 26 g protein

MCDONALD'S

EAT THIS!
Egg McMuffin

Per serving: 300 calories, 12 g fat (6 g saturated fat), 730 mg sodium, 29 g carbs, 2 g sugars, 1 g fiber, 17 g protein

NOT THAT!
Sausage Biscuit with Egg

Per serving: 510 calories, 33 g fat (14 g saturated fat), 1,170 mg sodium, 36 g carbs, 18 g protein

OLIVE GARDEN

EAT THIS!

Chicken Margherita

Per lunch portion: 370 calories, 22 g fat (7 g saturated fat, 0 g trans fat), 700 mg sodium, 8 g carbs, 2 g fiber, 3 g sugars, 37 g protein

NOT THAT!

Chicken & Shrimp Carbonara

Per serving: 1,390 calories, 94 g fat (50 g saturated fat, 3 g trans fat), 2,050 mg sodium, 75 g carbs, 10 g sugars, 3 g fiber, 64 g protein

ON THE BORDER

EAT THIS!

Grilled Fish Tacos Del Mar

Per serving: 320 calories, 14 g fat (1.5 g saturated fat), 690 mg sodium, 31 g carbs, 5 g sugars, 4 g fiber, 21 g protein

NOT THAT!

3 Sauce Fajita Burrito

Per serving: 900 calories, 40 g fat (18 g saturated fat), 4,370 mg sodium, 72 g carbs, 11 g sugars, 5 g fiber, 64 g protein

OUTBACK STEAKHOUSE

EAT THIS!

Victoria's 6-ounce Filet Mignon with sides of Asparagus and House Salad

Per serving: 388 calories, 18.9 g fat (7 g saturated fat, 0.7 g trans fat), n/a sodium, 15 g carbs, 5.2 g fiber, 42.7 g protein

NOT THAT!

Bloomin' Onion

Per serving: 1,950 calories, 155 g fat (56 g saturated fat, 7 g trans fat), 3,840 mg sodium, 123 g carbs, 18 g sugars, 14 g fiber, 18 g protein

PANDA EXPRESS

EAT THIS!

Broccoli Beef

Per serving: 150 calories, 7 g fat (1.5 g saturated fat), 520 mg sodium, 13 g carbs, 7 g sugars, 2 g fiber, 9 g protein

NOT THAT!

Black Pepper Chicken

Per serving: 280 calories, 19 g fat (1.5 g saturated fat), 1,130 mg sodium, 15 g carbs, 7 g sugars, 1 g fiber, 13 g protein

P.F. CHANG'S

EAT THIS!

Spicy Tuna Roll

Per serving: 300 calories, 6 g fat (1 g saturated fat), 670 mg sodium, 43 g carbs, 10 g sugars, 2 g fiber, 19 g protein

NOT THAT!

Hot and Sour Soup Bowl

Per serving: 470 calories, 12 g fat (2.5 g saturated fat), 3,800 mg sodium, 63 g carbs, 8 g sugars, 3 g fiber, 26 g protein

POPEYE'S

EAT THIS!

6 piece Handcrafted Nuggets

Per serving: 225 calories, 14 g fat (6 g saturated fat, 1 g trans fat), 345 mg sodium, 15 g carbs, 2 g fiber, 11 g protein

NOT THAT!

5 piece Handcrafted Tenders—Spicy or Mild

Per serving: 741 calories, 34 g fat (14 g saturated fat, 2 g trans fat), 3,035 mg sodium, 48 g carbs, 3 g fiber, 63 g protein

RED LOBSTER

EAT THIS!
Live Maine Lobster 1¼ lbs Stuffed

Per serving: 570 calories, 38 g fat (23 g saturated fat), 800 mg sodium, 2 g sugars, 44 g protein

NOT THAT!
Crispy Calamari and Vegetables

Per serving: 1,770 calories, 122 g fat (12 g saturated fat, 0.5 g trans fat), 4,570 mg sodium, 138 g carbs, 19 g sugars, 8 g fiber, 31 g protein

RED ROBIN

EAT THIS!
The Wedgie

Per serving: 500 calories, 30 g fat (10 g saturated fat, 1 g trans fat), 750 mg sodium, 23 g carbs, 13 g sugars, 8 g fiber, 37 g protein

NOT THAT!
Clucks & Fries Buffalo Style

Per serving: 1,620 calories, 114 g fat (28 g saturated fat, 1 g trans fat), 4,060 mg sodium, 103 g carbs, 3 g sugars, 18 g fiber, 48 g protein

SONIC

EAT THIS!
Original Pretzel Dog—6"

Per serving: 320 calories, 20 g fat (8 g saturated fat), 760 mg sodium, 23 g carbs, 2 g sugars, 11 g protein

NOT THAT!
Large Chili Cheese Tots

Per serving: 960 calories, 57 g fat (17 g saturated fat), 2,690 mg sodium, 92 g carb, 3 g sugars, 19 g protein

SUBWAY

EAT THIS!

6" Oven Roasted Chicken Sandwich

Per serving: 320 calories, 5 g fat (1.5 g saturated fat), 610 mg sodium, 46 g carbs, 8 g sugars, 5 g fiber, 23 g protein

NOT THAT!

Turkey, Bacon and Guacamole on Tomato Basil Wrap

Per serving: 810 calories, 42 g fat (13 g saturated fat, 0.5 g trans fat), 2,960 mg sodium, 62 g carbs, 6 g sugars, 5 g fiber, 43 g protein

TACO BELL

EAT THIS!

Chalupa Supreme—Steak

Per serving: 330 calories, 16 g fat (4 g saturated fat), 530 mg sodium, 32 g carbs, 3 g sugars, 2 g fiber, 15 g protein

NOT THAT!

XXL Grilled Stuft Chicken Burrito

Per serving: 870 calories, 40 g fat (14 g saturated fat, 1 g trans fat), 2,140 mg sodium, 97 g carbs, 6 g sugars, 13 g fiber, 32 g protein

WENDY'S

EAT THIS!

Grilled Chicken Sandwich

Per serving: 370 calories, 10 g fat (2 g saturated fat), 830 mg sodium, 38 g carbs, 8 g sugars, 3 g fiber, 34 g protein

NOT THAT!

Awesome Bacon Classic Triple

Per serving: 1,170 calories, 78 g fat (32 g saturated fat, 4 g trans fat), 1,930 mg sodium, 43 g carbs, 8 g sugars, 3 g fiber, 76 g protein